NCRP REPORT No. 155

Management of Radionuclide Therapy Patients

Recommendations of the
**NATIONAL COUNCIL ON RADIATION
PROTECTION AND MEASUREMENTS**

December 11, 2006

National Council on Radiation Protection and Measurements
7910 Woodmont Avenue, Suite 400 / Bethesda, MD 20814-3095

LEGAL NOTICE

Disclaimer

Library of Congress Cataloging-in-Publication Data

Management of radionuclide therapy patients.
    p. cm. — (NCRP report ; no. 155)
"December 11, 2006."
"Prepared by NCRP Scientific Committee 91-1 on Precautions in the Management of Patients Who Have Received Therapeutic Amounts of Radioactivity"--Pref.
Supersedes NCRP Report No. 37, Precautions in the Management of Patients Who Have Received Therapeutic Amounts of Radionuclides, 1970.
Includes bibliographical references and index.
ISBN-13: 978-0-929600-92-5
ISBN-10: 0-929600-92-4
    1. Radiotherapy--Standards--United States. 2. Radiotherapy--United States--Safety measures. 3. Radiation--Safety regulations--United States I. National Council on Radiation Protection and Measurements. II. National Council on Radiation Protection and Measurements. Scientific Committee 91-1 on Precautions in the Management of Patients Who Have Received Therapeutic Amounts of Radioactivity. III. Series.
    [DNLM: 1. Radiotherapy--standards--Guideline. 2. Radiation Injuries--prevention & control--Guideline. 3. Radiation Protection--methods--Guideline.
WN 250 M266 2007]
    RM854.M36 2007
    615.8'42--dc22

                      2007010967

[For detailed information on the availability of NCRP publications see page 234.]

Preface

This Report was developed under the auspices of Program Area Committee 4 of the National Council on Radiation Protection and Measurements (NCRP) concerned with radiation protection in medicine. The Report supersedes NCRP Report No. 37, *Precautions in the Management of Patients Who Have Received Therapeutic Amounts of Radionuclides*, which was issued in 1970. Thus, this Report addresses the current issues and practices that have developed during the long period before this updating. The Report provides radiation protection guidance for physicians, medical physicists, health physicists, nuclear pharmacists, health care professionals, and visitors to medical facilities, family members of the patients as well as members of the public who may be involved in the treatment and care of radionuclide therapy patients. This Report also confirms the recommendations of NCRP Commentary No. 11 on *Dose Limits for Individuals Who Receive Exposure from Radionuclide Therapy Patients*, and confirms or updates related recommendations in other earlier NCRP publications identified in Section 1 of this Report.

Throughout the Report amounts of activity are stated for the practices or procedures under discussion. This is done only for illustration purposes and these amounts are not to be taken as actual prescriptions for the particular practices or procedures. The prescription of activity for a patient is the sole responsibility of the prescribing physician.

This Report is dedicated to Dr. John S. Laughlin of the Memorial Sloan-Kettering Cancer Center, a pioneer in the field of medical physics, who contributed to many advancements in the treatment of cancer, and who was a member of the Scientific Committee that produced the first report issued in 1970 and who died in late 2004.

This Report was prepared by NCRP Scientific Committee 91-1 on Precautions in the Management of Patients Who Have Received Therapeutic Amounts of Radioactivity. Serving on Scientific Committee 91-1 were:

Jean St. Germain, *Chairman*
Memorial Sloan-Kettering Cancer Center
New York, New York

iii

Members

Edward B. Silberstein
University of Cincinnati
   Medical Center
Cincinnati, Ohio

Richard J. Vetter
Mayo Clinic
Rochester, Minnesota

Jeffrey F. Williamson
Washington University
   Medical Center
St. Louis, Missouri

Pat D. Zanzonico
Memorial Sloan-Kettering
   Cancer Center
New York, New York

Liaisons

Jerrold T. Bushberg
University of California,
   Davis School of Medicine
Sacramento, California

Sarah S. Donaldson
Stanford University School
   of Medicine
Stanford, California

NCRP Secretariat
Constantine J. Maletskos, *Staff Consultant*, 2003–2006
William M. Beckner, *Senior Staff Scientist*, 2001–2003
James A. Spahn, Jr., *Senior Staff Scientist*, 1994–2000
Cindy L. O'Brien, *Managing Editor*
David A. Schauer, *Executive Director*

The Council wishes to express its appreciation to the Committee members, liaisons and consultants for the time and effort devoted to the preparation of this Report.

Financial support was provided by the U.S. Nuclear Regulatory Commission (NRC) and the National Cancer Institute (NCI Contract #2 R24 CA 074296-09A1). The contents of this Report are the sole responsibility of NCRP, and do not necessarily represent the official views of NRC or the NCI, National Institutes of Health.

Thomas S. Tenforde
President

Contents

Executive Summary

This Report is intended for use by a wide readership including physicians, medical physicists, health physicists, administrators, nurses, other professional and medical staff, and patients.[1] The approaches originally suggested in NCRP Report No. 37, *Precautions in the Management of Patients Who Have Received Therapeutic Amounts of Radionuclides*, are incorporated and updated (NCRP, 1970).

There are aspects of this Report that will, of necessity, touch on the physician-patient relationship. The requirements to explain risks from therapeutic procedures and to obtain adequate, informed patient consent are proper roles of the treating physician and the institutional review board of the facility involved. It is within the charge of the institutional review board as defined in federal regulations to review the propriety and language of consent forms; to judge the understanding of the content of consent forms and investigative protocols by the patient, the patient's representative or family; and to judge the adequacy of statements about radiation risk. In many facilities, the radiation safety committee (RSC) is advisory to the institutional review board in making this judgment. A discussion of risks associated with radiation doses and informed consent is beyond the scope of this Report. Information about radiation risks is available in NCRP Report No. 115 (NCRP, 1993a) and other publications cited in the references.

NCRP made an arbitrary division between sealed and unsealed radioactive sources and considered all unsealed sources under the category of radiopharmaceutical therapy, although some unsealed source applications will fit the category of device as defined by the U.S. Food and Drug Administration (FDA). Sealed radioactive sources are considered in the brachytherapy section. Depending on the ethos of a particular facility, the lines of this division may blur, however the particular recommendations would still apply.

---

[1]In some parts of the Report, the reader will find both International System (SI) units and conventional units (*e.g.*, curie). This approach reflects the current state of medical practice in making the transition to the SI system in the United States.

1

Section 1 of this Report is an introduction and includes some brief historical items. This Section discusses the basic principles of both radiopharmaceutical therapy and brachytherapy. Section 2 deals with basic radiation safety principles in a medical facility and includes a description of the radiation safety program, dose limits, staffing and definitions specific to this Report. Section 3 addresses radiopharmaceutical therapy including both clinical and radiation safety aspects. Appendices A and B expand on the patient-release criteria outlined in Section 3 and include a spreadsheet program for assisting in determining patient-release instructions. Section 4 deals specifically with brachytherapy including techniques, terminology, and a brief discussion of applicable dosimetry. Appendix C presents a discussion of quality-assurance (QA) requirements for high dose-rate (HDR) afterloading which is an increasingly useful modality. Appendix D outlines shielding requirements for HDR brachytherapy installations.

Both Sections 3 and 4 discuss radiation doses and administered activity levels. The actual activities or radiation doses used for any individual patient will be prescribed by the treating physician and may vary considerably from the amounts shown. The radiation doses or administered activities listed are only an indication of what may be used. The amounts listed are not a substitute for an individual prescription, and this Report is not a prescribing manual. Any of the numerical values used for illustration of processes or examples involved are not recommendations.

Section 5 includes facility design for both nuclear-medicine and radiation-oncology installations. Section 6 describes changes in patients' status, including medical emergencies and presents guidelines for other situations that may be adapted to readers' facilities.

Dose Limits

Due to the infrequent nature of potential radiation exposures and because of the substantial benefits that accrue to the family from a patient's treatment, a radiation dose limit of 5 mSv annually for members of the patient's family is recommended. This recommendation is consistent with the recommendations of NCRP Commentary No. 11 (NCRP, 1995a).

Patient Confinement

Medical confinement in a hospital or skilled-care facility of a patient receiving radionuclide therapeutic treatment is intended to minimize the radiation dose to the public and to members of the patient's family. Such treatment may range from oral ingestion of a capsule containing radioactive material to emplacement of sealed sources by a surgical procedure. However, it is recognized that the presence and support of a patient's family may contribute substantially to the therapeutic outcome and improve the patient's quality-of-life. The treating physician, in consultation with the facility radiation safety officer (RSO), will determine the need for medical confinement. This decision will consider the physical and mental condition of the patient as well as the individual living circumstances. It should be possible for the majority of patients to be treated as outpatients if provided with adequate instructions, both oral and written, for the patient and his family, for other institutions with which the patient may interact, and for regulatory authorities.

Patient Records

Patient records, whether in written or electronic form, *should* clearly identify the radionuclide therapy procedure performed including the radionuclide and activity used as well as the physical and chemical form, the treating physician, and contact information. These records *should* be maintained in the records of the facility either permanently or for a time designated by the relevant regulatory agencies.

NCRP recognizes that there are existing federal or state regulatory requirements covering many topics in this Report and the recommendations in this Report are not intended to supplant these regulations. These regulations, where applicable, *should* be consulted in applying the general principles discussed. However, NCRP considered that it had a broader mandate than to simply recapitulate regulations. As a particular example, NCRP reviewed the regulatory definitions of "misadministration" and "medical events" and chose to define an alternate term, "addressable events," that included the regulatory requirements, but expanded consideration to include events that may have systematic implications. Therefore, addressable events as defined will include events that could result in patient injury or harm as well as events that have no associated injury. The intent of the term, addressable events, is to indicate a broader mandate to examine the cause of an event, systematic changes as required, and any necessary changes in practice.

The rapid advance of technology and the enlarging field of radionuclide applications will cause some of the specific treatments in this Report to eventually become outdated. However, the basic principles discussed and the radiation protection guidelines presented should remain constant.

1. Introduction

The treatment of cancer and certain other allied diseases relies on the use of ionizing radiation or radionuclides in various modalities. The use of high-energy x rays and electrons is reserved to external-beam radiotherapy (ERT) and the field of radiation oncology. Patients treated with ERT do not represent a hazard to staff or family and are not the subject of this Report. The use of unsealed radionuclides for radiopharmaceutical therapy falls to the practice of nuclear medicine. The use of sealed radionuclides for brachytherapy falls to the practice of radiation oncology. Together, these fields form the substance of this Report and are collectively identified in this Report as radionuclide therapy.

The approaches originally suggested in NCRP Report No. 37, *Precautions in the Management of Patients Who Have Received Therapeutic Amounts of Radionuclides*, are incorporated and updated (NCRP, 1970). NCRP Report No. 124, *Sources and Magnitude of Occupational and Public Exposures from Nuclear Medicine Procedures*, discusses the magnitude of occupational and public exposures from nuclear-medicine procedures and is a companion report (NCRP, 1996). This Report also incorporates discussions found in NCRP Report No. 105, *Radiation Protection for Medical and Allied Health Personnel*; NCRP Report No. 127, *Operational Radiation Safety Program*; as well as recommendations discussed in NCRP Commentary No. 9, *Considerations Regarding the Unintended Radiation Exposure of the Embryo, Fetus or Nursing Child*; NCRP Commentary No. 11, *Dose Limits for Individuals Who Receive Exposure from Radionuclide Therapy Patients*; and NCRP Statement No. 10, *Recent Applications of the NCRP Public Dose Limit Recommendation for Ionizing Radiation* (NCRP, 1989; 1994; 1995a; 1998; 2004a). In addition, NCRP Annual Meeting Proceedings No. 19, *The Effects of Pre- and Postconception Exposure to Radiation*, and No. 21, *Radiation Protection in Medicine: Contemporary Issues*, cover several specific issues in a comprehensive format beyond the scope of this Report (NCRP, 1999a; 1999b).

This introduction outlines the principles within which NCRP framed its recommendations. Of necessity, NCRP could not deal with every conceivable situation or application. However, the general guidelines stated and the overall philosophy presented *should*

4

provide a template for a medical facility seeking to administer therapeutic amounts of radionuclides to patients needing such services while providing a safe working environment for other patients, medical staff, family members, visitors, and the public.

Throughout the Report amounts of activity are stated for the practices or procedures under discussion. This is done only for illustration purposes and these amounts are not to be taken as actual prescriptions for the particular practices or procedures. The prescription of activity for a patient is the sole responsibility of the prescribing physician.

Terms and symbols used in this Report are defined in the text and in the Glossary. Recommendations throughout this Report are expressed in terms of *shall* and *should* (in italics) where:

- *shall* indicates a recommendation that is necessary to meet currently accepted standards of radiation protection; and
- *should* indicates an advisory recommendation that is to be applied when practicable or practical (*e.g.*, cost effective).

1.1 Brief History

It seems appropriate at the beginning of the 21st century to mention, albeit briefly, some landmarks in the history of therapeutic radiation applications, particularly in view of four recent centennials (*i.e.*, the 1995 centennial of the discovery of x rays, the 1998 centennial of the discovery of radium, the 2003 centennial of the award of the Nobel Prize to Marie Curie and Henri Becquerel, and the 2005 centennial of the publications by Albert Einstein on the theory of relativity). For those persons wishing to explore this fascinating history in more depth, a number of references are provided (Curie, 1938; del Regato, 1985; 1996a; 1996b; Quimby, 1948).

The discovery of x rays by Wilhelm Conrad Roentgen in 1895 appeared in all of the news media of his day (Dam, 1896). In 1896, Emil Grubbe started radiation treatments for a postoperative recurrence of breast cancer, the first attempt at radiotherapy anywhere in the world (del Regato, 1996a). Within the first year following Roentgen's discovery, almost 1,000 papers were published on applications of x rays. The problems of tube design limited early tubes to the production of x rays with voltages close to 60 kV, suitable for treatment in dermatology. In 1914, William D. Coolidge published his paper describing the first successful roentgen-ray tube built with a tungsten filament (Coolidge, 1913). This discovery made possible the use of x rays of the order of 200 kV, so called "deep therapy."

In 1896, the eminent French scientist, Henri Becquerel, first detected naturally occurring radioactive substances and suggested that the study of this phenomenon might prove an interesting doctoral thesis for Marie Curie. The work of Marie and Pierre Curie began in a search for the properties of radioactive materials, and finally resulted in experiments on thorium (Curie, 1938). Testing of pitchblende ores secured from the mines of Joachimsthal showed higher levels of activity than were predicted for thorium alone. Madame Curie's search for a new element resulted in the discovery of polonium in 1898, named for her native Poland (Curie, 1938). Further refinement of this ore resulted in the discovery of a second radioactive element, radium (Curie et al., 1898). Both discoveries began to be used immediately in medicine (Curie, 1938; Glasser, 1961).

In 1905, Robert Abbe attempted the first interstitial application in the United States (del Regato, 1996a). The Pasteur Laboratory of the Radium Institute at the University of Paris was founded in 1909. After World War I, the team of George Richard, Jean Pierquin, and Octave Monod began therapeutic trials to develop treatment methods for radium (del Regato, 1996a).

Abbe initiated a procedure in which tubes of radium were left post-operatively in the vicinity of tumors, the predecessor of modern afterloading techniques (del Regato, 1996a). Radium ore imported from Africa or Eastern Europe was a scarce and costly commodity. American mines in Colorado were opened to allow American hospitals to obtain radium at lower but still significant costs (del Regato, 1996a). William Duane, who had studied with Marie Curie in Paris for several years, developed a radium emanation and extraction process. In 1917, Duane installed a radon plant at the Memorial Hospital in New York City. Radon was captured in glass capillary tubes that could be cut into sections, "seeds," to be brought into contact with tumors (Brucer, 1993). Duane's methods were improved upon by Gioacchino Failla, who had also studied with Marie Curie. Failla's improvements included placing the radon into gold capillary tubes, adding the advantage of filtration (del Regato, 1996a). Claudius Regaud demonstrated experimentally that a moderate total dose of radiation subdivided into fractions and administered in several exposures was more effective than a single large dose (del Regato, 1996a). Fractionated dose regimens were elaborated by Edith Quimby at the Memorial Hospital who developed treatment schemes for irradiation (Quimby, 1931; 1935; 1937; 1948). In 1938, only 39 American physicians confined their practice to therapeutic radiology and most of these physicians had been self-taught or received training in Europe (del Regato,

1996b). The development of radiation oncology as a specialty is addressed in several publications, notably the historical articles published by del Regato (1996a; 1996b). By 1940, commercial x-ray units of one or two million volts were available in the United States. However, there were physicians and physicists who favored the use of radium sources to deliver doses exterior to the body, so-called teletherapy. A teletherapy unit using 4 g of radium was installed and built at the Memorial Hospital. However, the clinical results were not sufficiently impressive to justify continued use.

During the 1930s, Edith Quimby published tables for the calculation of doses from implants in tissues and investigated the use of various sources in interstitial therapy (Quimby, 1931; 1935). Paterson and Parker presented refined calculation systems for delivering uniform doses to implanted volumes (Paterson, 1934; Paterson et al., 1936). In 1958, Ulrich Henschke used ^{192}Ir seeds for temporary implants and began using afterloading techniques for brachytherapy. Refinements led to the introduction of remote afterloading in the 1960s (Henschke, 1963). Also, in the 1960s, a number of radium/radon substitute sources were investigated and in 1965, the first implant using ^{125}I seeds was performed at the Memorial Hospital (Hilaris, 1975). In the 1980s, ^{103}Pd seeds became available and were used for interstitial procedures.

1.2 Research with Radioactive Material

In 1923, George de Hevesy studied plant metabolism with ^{212}Pb and developed the concept of radioactive tracers. He also performed the first radioactive trace studies in animals during the following years and published his results in 1948 (de Hevesy, 1948).

In 1934, Frederic Joliot and Irene Curie published a paper that described the first chemical proof of artificial transmutation as well as demonstrating that an alpha particle was captured in these reactions (Joliot and Curie, 1934). The transmutation of beryllium, magnesium and aluminum gave birth to new species that emitted positrons (e.g., ^{13}N). This paper, in <600 words, described the process for making these new isotopes that would later have application in nuclear medicine. This discovery would bring the authors a Nobel Prize.

The announcement from the Manhattan Project of the availability of large quantities of various artificially-produced radionuclides ushered in a new era of medical research (Manhattan, 1946). Cobalt-60 was one of the first radionuclides investigated because of its relatively long half-life and potential for use in therapeutic applications (Myers, 1948). Three-hundred shipments of various artificial radionuclides were made during the first year of operation. By 1956, the number of shipments had risen to 15,000 and 5,000 institutions were placing orders (Quimby, 1970).

First produced in minute quantities by George de Hevesy in 1934, ^{32}P, as sodium phosphate, became an obvious therapeutic choice to treat a variety of neoplasias when Ernest Lawrence's cyclotron at the University of California, Berkeley, could produce significant quantities of the radionuclide (de Hevesy, 1948). Ernest's brother, a physician, John Lawrence, reported partial responses to ^{32}P in chronic myelogenous leukemia by 1938, while Lowell Erf and others at Berkeley found ^{32}P effective in treating *polycythemia vera* by 1941. Meanwhile a joint program at Massachusetts General Hospital and the Massachusetts Institute of Technology, begun in 1937, focused on radioiodine for thyroid diseases. The first radioiodine produced, in April 1937, was ^{128}I, which had a very short half-life, <30 min, but allowed for basic physiological studies. The progress by Glenn Seaborg and John Livingood at Berkeley to discover longer-lived iodine radioisotopes was rapid, and the first article on ^{131}I, with an 8 d half-life, appeared only 30 months later, in October 1939. In two more years a patient had been scanned for metastases from thyroid cancer with radioiodine, but World War II caused a hiatus in research with medical uses of radionuclides. In 1946, Samuel Seidlin announced the first cure of thyroid cancer with ^{131}I. In the decade following the end of World War II, iodine labeling of human albumin allowed study of the blood pool and detection of brain tumors, iodinated rose bengal was used to study liver physiology and anatomy, and radioiron production led to detailed studies of erythropoiesis.

At the University of California Berkeley, Ernest Lawrence designed the first cyclotron and produced radionuclides by bombardment with accelerated particles (Lawrence, 1934; 1936). Lawrence received the Nobel Prize in 1939 for this development. The use of cyclotrons for radionuclide production reduced the dependence on reactor-produced sources and allowed for the production of short-lived positron-emitting radionuclides and other radionuclides not made in reactors.

The development of the molybdenum/technetium generator in the 1970s provided the stimulus for the synthesis of many new radiopharmaceuticals. The production of the parent element, ^{99}Mo, was a reactor-based operation, but the availability of the short-lived ^{99m}Tc decay product allowed larger activities to be administered to patients with lower radiation doses compared to previously used radionuclides. Technetium-99m labeled compounds replaced older tracers such as ^{203}Hg and ^{197}Hg for renal studies and the use of ^{198}Au colloid for liver imaging. By the end of the 20th century, ~80 % of diagnostic nuclear-medicine procedures were performed with ^{99m}Tc.

In the late 1960s, the availability of cyclotrons small enough to be placed in medical centers made possible the exploration of the use of positron-emitting isotopes such as ^{18}F, ^{11}C, and ^{15}O for diagnostic nuclear-medicine studies. The full diagnostic capabilities of positron-labeled pharmaceuticals, such as ^{18}F-fluorodeoxyglucose, in the fields of neurologic and oncologic imaging were finally realized in the 1990s due to improvements in imaging technology. The use of ^{18}F-fluorodeoxyglucose, a tracer of glucose metabolism, to measure localized increase in glucose metabolism has provided a unique insight into the detection and staging of a variety of cancers (Hustinx *et al.*, 1996).

1.3 Principles of Radiopharmaceutical Therapy

The major objective of radiopharmaceutical therapy has been to maximize the uptake and retention of activity in a target organ, especially an organ containing a tumor, while minimizing the uptake of activity in normal tissue. Tissue uptake and retention is controlled by the chemical and physical properties of the radiopharmaceutical. Therapeutic radiopharmaceuticals are employed in anticipation of a selective tumoricidal effect on the target tissue. As opposed to ERT where the radiation must pass through some normal tissue, the orally or intravenously administered radiopharmaceuticals currently employed have a relatively selective uptake in malignant tissue. Among the essential properties of therapeutic radionuclides are charged particle emissions (*e.g.*, alpha or electron emissions), a high ratio of charged particle to photon energy abundance, and if possible, a physical half-life substantially longer than the exponential or nearly exponential rise of the administered activity in a particular organ or tissue and substantially shorter than the biological half-life of the radiopharmaceutical in the target tissue. These properties are intended to increase the ratio of radiation dose delivered to the target tumor to the radiation dose received by the rest of the body. The majority of therapeutic radiopharmaceuticals in use today emit beta particles of sufficient energy to traverse many layers of tumor cells adjacent to the deposition of the pharmaceutical. For micrometastases, radionuclides that emit Auger electrons with relatively short path lengths or alpha particles that can traverse two or three cell diameters before dissipating their energy may be desirable. Criteria for radionuclide selection are discussed in Section 3.

Radionuclide localization techniques have involved approaches such as the use of hormone receptors (*e.g.*, somatostatin) tumor antigens of varying specificity reacting with labeled antibodies; and uptakes of radiotracers that are incorporated into specific physiological processes [*e.g.*, sodium iodide (Na^{131}I)]. Several approaches have been attempted to reduce uptake in nontarget tissue. These approaches have involved enhancing excretion from the bladder, bowel and salivary glands in order to markedly reduce radiation toxicity to these organs. Other techniques involve the administration of nonlabeled pharmaceuticals, so-called blocking doses, that are intended to prevent uptake in the primary site that is not the object of the treatment and, therefore, force the radiopharmaceutical to be concentrated in a secondary site.

1.4 Principles of Brachytherapy

The name, brachytherapy, derives from the Greek prefix, "brachys," meaning short, literally therapy at short distances. The term is generally understood to mean the placement of sealed sources within or adjacent to a treatment site. This technique requires that the area to be treated be accessible and that the tumor be geometrically limited and be of small to moderate size. Access will generally involve some type of surgical intervention. The tumor will be subjected to continuous irradiation to a total prescribed therapeutic dose for as long as the sources are present. Brachytherapy may be the primary treatment or be an adjunct (*i.e.*, a "boost") to ERT.

Sealed sources may be left in place permanently, as in interstitial seed implants, or placed temporarily and removed after a prescribed treatment time, such as in intracavitary treatment. Determination as to whether a radionuclide is suitable for permanent or temporary use is usually a function of the half-life of the source. In general, ^{125}I with a half-life equal to 60 d is the longest lived radionuclide used for permanent implants. In temporary implantation, sources may be placed within an applicator that has been placed in a body cavity, within catheters that have been placed in or around a tumor, and plaques placed on the skin or mucosal surface. Criteria for source selection are discussed in Section 4.

The most frequent use of temporary implantation is for the treatment of gynecological tumors. The techniques initially developed for gynecological applications involved the use of applicators into which the sealed sources had been loaded prior to placement, so-called "preloaded" applications. The applicator, loaded with sealed sources, was brought to the operating room. The loaded applicator was placed within the body cavity and manually manipulated into the correct position by the physician. A technique was also available for placement of sealed sources within the uterine cavity, a technique known as Heyman packing. This technique relied on manual positioning of the sources. Both of these techniques involved doses to everyone within the operating room and recovery areas and resulted in large doses to the treating physician, typically a surgeon or gynecologist. These techniques were replaced in the period from the 1960s to the 1970s by afterloading techniques in which sources are positioned at some time following the placement of the source holder, typically a catheter. In afterloading, there are no doses received by the surgical or recovery staff because the sealed sources are positioned after the surgical intervention and treatment plan. The treating physician was typically a radiologist or radiation oncologist.

Another brachytherapy technique involves the placement of sources, either permanently or temporarily, within interstitial spaces. For temporary implants, sources were fashioned into needles for direct insertion into tissue or placement in catheters during a surgical procedure. One of the first radionuclides used for seed implantation was ^{222}Rn. These seeds were manufactured by the capture of radon gas in gold seeds. Another early technique intended to replace the use of radon seeds involved the use of ^{198}Au seeds, originally called gold grains to distinguish these seeds from the ^{222}Rn seeds (Sinclair, 1952). The accumulated therapeutic experience prior to 1960 relied on the use of radium and radon sources. The use of radium-substitute sources, such as ^{60}Co or ^{137}Cs, became possible after reactor-produced sources became available. In the 1960s, ^{192}Ir sources were introduced and techniques using these sources remain in current use (Henschke, 1963). Temporary interstitial treatment techniques using high-specific activity sources of ^{125}I [i.e., 185 to 1,850 MBq (5 to 10 mCi)] were developed because their use offered significant radiation protection advantages. However, due to cost, these sources have not found wide acceptance. Interstitial techniques may involve the permanent placement of small sealed sources, "seeds," within the tumor itself. The seeds are introduced into tissue using either needle placement or "guns" that can place multiple seeds along a plane within the tumor volume (Hodt et al., 1952). The most common use of this technique is in prostrate brachytherapy with the seeds implanted through the perineum under imaging guidance. The possible radiobiological advantages of various techniques and sources have been discussed (Ling, 1992).

In brachytherapy, a small volume of tissue can be treated at dose levels higher than the doses delivered by conventional external-beam techniques. The isodose lines exhibit a higher dose gradient and, therefore, the treatment volume needs to be carefully defined. In a certain sense, brachytherapy techniques represent the ultimate in conformal therapy. Many of the techniques described in Section 4 involve some surgical intervention, which may not be suitable for all patients.

1.5 General Considerations

Radiopharmaceutical therapy and brachytherapy *should* be specifically planned for each individual so that therapeutic objectives are achieved with minimum irradiation of both the patient and hospital personnel. It is the responsibility of the treating physician (*e.g.*, the nuclear-medicine physician or radiation oncologist) to ensure that all pertinent information is available so that the therapeutic procedure can be justified and optimized. Available information *should* include consideration of alternative treatments, the risks and relative efficacy of all treatments, and also the impact of radiopharmaceutical therapy and brachytherapy, including medical confinement and post-release radiation precautions, on the overall well being of the patient. Patients and families *should* be provided with informational materials that are both comprehensive and easy to understand. Where appropriate, such materials *should* also be available for non-English speaking populations. If there is a choice of radiopharmaceuticals available for a therapy procedure, the relative merits of the chemical, biological and physical properties of each pharmaceutical in terms of reduction of radiation risks *should* be considered. Availability, relative costs, and other logistical issues may also affect the treatment decision.

Patient age and lifestyle-related issues will influence the consideration of treatment modality. For example, for a younger person wishing to start a family in the near or distant future, the possible consequences of significant gonadal irradiation incidental to radiopharmaceutical therapy or brachytherapy *should* be considered and discussed with the patient. The long-term reproductive consequences of high activity radionuclide therapy as well as any possible short-term impairment of fertility following such therapy may be of concern to the patient. In women of childbearing age, the possibility of pregnancy at the time of treatment and the justification for the procedure *shall* be carefully and explicitly considered. Whether female patients are breastfeeding small children *shall* also be explicitly considered for radiopharmaceutical therapy.

The pediatric patient is also of special concern, not only because of the generally greater radiation sensitivity of rapidly dividing cells but also because of the longer period of risk for radiogenic sequelae following therapy. While radiopharmaceutical therapy or brachytherapy in children is relatively rare, such therapies may well be critical for the patient. The biological distribution, metabolism and excretion of radiopharmaceuticals vary widely with age, and differences are most pronounced in infancy and old age. Therefore, age-dependent dosimetry models *should* be used in planning radiopharmaceutical therapy.

For all therapeutic administrations, an appropriate entry *shall* be made in the patients' medical records which includes the date and time of therapy, the activity used and the identity of the radionuclide. For radiopharmaceutical therapy, this information *shall* also include the radiopharmaceutical and the date and time of assay. Medical facilities undertaking any form of therapy involving the therapeutic applications of radionuclides *shall* have a QA program in place. The details of these programs and specifics of radionuclide administrations are discussed in the following sections.

2. Radiation Safety Program in a Medical Facility

This Section describes the controls (administrative, procedural and engineered) necessary for a radiation safety program in a medical facility that utilizes therapeutic quantities of radionuclides. The discussion provided in this Section is not intended to cover all situations encountered in every type of medical facility. It should be considered as guidance to assist the facility in developing its own procedures and QA program. Additional guidance may be found in other NCRP reports and International Commission on Radiological Protection (ICRP) publications (ICRP, 1983; 1989; NCRP, 1983; 1989; 1995b; 1998). Various scientific organizations have addressed topics covered in this Report and have published task group reports or specific guidance. These organizations include, among others, the American Association of Physicists in Medicine (AAPM), American College of Radiology, American College of Medical Physics, Health Physics Society, and the Society of Nuclear Medicine. A number of these reports are included in the references of this Report. However, a complete listing may be found on the websites of the various organizations.

2.1 Description of the Radiation Safety Program

Medical facilities that use sealed and unsealed radioactive sources for therapeutic purposes *shall* have a radiation safety program. The program *shall* be commensurate with the hazards associated with use of the radioactive sources and *shall* adequately protect workers and the public. Prior to the use of any radioactive source, facility management or an appropriate physician or physicist *shall* consult with a qualified expert[2] to evaluate the potential radiation hazards and to develop appropriate elements of the radiation safety program. The radiation safety program *shall* be

---

[2]Qualified expert is defined in the Glossary and the sections that follow.

reviewed annually to confirm that it continues to meet the operational objectives of the facility, the recommendations of appropriate standards and the requirements of federal, state and local regulations. The annual review *shall* be conducted by a qualified expert who has similar program experience. The qualified expert for these activities may be an individual who works for the facility or an outside expert. The program *shall* include appropriate policies, practices and equipment to maintain radiation exposures to workers and the public as low as reasonably achievable (ALARA), social and economic factors being taken into account.

A facility Radiation Safety Officer (RSO) *shall* be designated to fulfill the responsibilities described in Section 2.3.2. In small programs the RSO may be a physician or physicist knowledgeable in radiation safety practice. The qualifications for the RSO will depend on the size and complexity of the facility, but the RSO *shall* have appropriate education, training and experience to adequately address the needs of the program. Large, complex practices *should* consider requiring the RSO to be certified by a specialty board such as the American Board of Health Physics, the American Board of Medical Physics, the American Board of Radiology, or the American Board of Nuclear Medicine. The RSO *should* seek advice from other qualified experts, as necessary, whenever the facility considers use of a new modality or new radiation source that has characteristics different from those currently in use.

2.2 Current Dose Limits and Radiation Protection Goals

2.2.1 *Recommended Dose Limits*

Current radiation protection standards are based on the assumption that any radiation dose above natural background may create some additional risk of damage, particularly cancer. Radiation protection is concerned with the total detriment from radiation exposure, which includes fatal and nonfatal cancers, hereditary defects, and potential life-span shortening. Thus, it is prudent to design a radiation safety program that maintains radiation doses to workers and the public ALARA.

The 1977 report of the United Nations Scientific Committee on the Effects of Atomic Radiation (UNSCEAR) was the first report in a series to provide risk estimates for cancer in a number of organs (UNSCEAR, 1977). The risk estimates were derived from a variety of studies but relied primarily on the data from the Japanese atomic-bomb survivors. The 1988 UNSCEAR report, the tenth in that series, revised the estimates from the 1977 report and considered excess cancer mortality as the major factor to be used in setting radiation protection standards (UNSCEAR, 1988). In 1990, the National Academy of Sciences/National Research Council (NAS/NRC) issued the Biological Effects of Ionizing Radiation (BEIR V) report (NAS/NRC, 1990) which updated earlier estimates of both the somatic and genetic effects of radiation and incorporated the estimates from the UNSCEAR (1988) report. Rates of mortality from various forms of cancer were analyzed in relation to age at irradiation, sex, time after irradiation, and other variables. In 2006, NAS/NRC issued BEIR VII (NAS/NRC, 2006) to update BEIR V using new information from epidemiologic and experimental research that accumulated since the 1990 review (NAS/NRC, 2006).

NCRP Report No. 91 (NCRP, 1987), now superseded by Report No. 116 (NCRP, 1993b), was the first in a series of reports that based radiation exposure limits on risk estimates. NCRP Report No. 115 (NCRP, 1993a) reviewed the risk estimates for radiation protection in light of the UNSCEAR (1988) report and BEIR V (NAS/NRC, 1990) report. This report provided the theoretical basis for the recommendations published in NCRP Report No. 116 (NCRP, 1993b). These recommendations for limitations of radiation exposure were established at a level to achieve the objectives of radiation protection (*i.e.*, prevention of the occurrence of clinically significant acute radiation damage and limitation of the risk of stochastic effects) such as cancer and genetic effects, and of deterministic effects, such as cataract induction. The risk estimates for radiation protection are discussed in NCRP Report No. 115 (NCRP, 1993a). These recommended limits for occupational dose and dose to members of the public are shown in Table 2.1 and exclude radiation doses received by an individual as a patient and doses from natural background radiation including radon. The risk associated with exposure to radiation doses within these limits is considered to be very small. However, it is assumed that increase in risk is proportional to dose; thus, NCRP recommends that the radiation safety program *shall* be designed to keep radiation doses ALARA.

The specific objectives of radiation protection as stated in NCRP Report No. 116 are:

- prevention of the occurrence of clinically significant radiation-induced deterministic effects by adhering to dose limits that are below the apparent threshold levels; and
- limitation of the risk of stochastic effects, cancer and genetic effects, to a reasonable level in relation to societal needs, values, benefits gained, and economic factors.

TABLE 2.1—*Recommended dose limits.*

Annual Effective Dose Limit (mSv)	
Adult workers[a]	50
Adult worker who declares her pregnancy[a]	0.5 mSv month^{-1}
Members of the public[a]	1
Family member of patient[b]	5
Pregnant women and children[b]	1
Trained and monitored family member of patient[b]	50
Adult lifetime[a]	Age × 10 mSv

[a]This Table affirms the recommendations of NCRP as published in Report No. 116 (NCRP, 1993b). Although these recommendations may be incorporated into regulation, they are not necessarily exactly the same as the dose limits that may be found in federal or state regulations (NRC, 1988). The references provided in the various sections of this Report may provide additional guidance.
[b]NCRP Commentary No. 11 and Statement No. 10 (NCRP, 1995a; 2004a).

NCRP Report No. 116 recommends that:

- any activity that involves radiation exposure *shall* be justified on the basis that the expected benefits to society exceed the overall societal cost (justification);
- the total societal detriment from justified activities or practices *shall* be maintained ALARA, economic and societal factors being taken into account; and
- individual dose limits *shall* be applied to ensure that the procedures of justification and ALARA do not result in individuals or groups of individuals exceeding levels of acceptable risk (limitation).

2.2.2 *Specific Definitions*

This Section provides some specific definitions used in later sections of this Report. Some of these definitions are specific to the medical care environment and others are defined in terms of a general understanding of the application of societal concepts within the medical environment. A Glossary is included in this Report for further information.

For purposes of limiting radiation doses, members of a patient's family *should* be considered as distinct from members of the public. However, for pregnant women and children who may be family members, the public limit would still apply. Typically, when a patient is diagnosed with a potentially life-threatening disease, such as cancer, the patient as well as members of the family are deeply affected. In such cases, judgments on the benefits to the patient and the family from family interactions need to be considered in the decisions on radiation protection standards.

A "family member" is any person who provides support and comfort to a patient on a regular basis and is considered by the patient as a member of their "family" whether by birth or marriage or by virtue of a close, loving relationship.

In some cases involving radiopharmaceutical therapy or brachytherapy, the patient *shall* be confined for purposes of radiation protection following the administration or emplacement of radioactive sources. This confinement *shall* take place within a "medical facility."

A "medical facility" is a hospital, clinic or other facility that may practice radiopharmaceutical therapy or brachytherapy and that provides in-patient care. This definition specifically excludes the patient's own home.

A radiopharmaceutical is any radioactive material in various forms that is administered to a patient *via* various routes so that the material is metabolized by the patient for distribution to various organs or tissues or the whole body for purposes of therapy. A radiopharmaceutical most often includes a radionuclide chemically bound to a reagent or carrier that localizes the radionuclide in specific organ systems or local lesions.

Members of the public, such as visitors to a medical facility may be in the vicinity of patients receiving radiation therapy. A "member of the public" is any adult person (*i.e.*, a person >18 y of age) not a member of the patient's family and not an individual exposed to radiation in the course of their employment as a result of the care and management of the patient.

Whether in written or electronic (computerized) form, a medical record, treatment folder or "chart" of a patient is the permanent institutional document in a medical facility that fully describes the medical history and care of the patient. Pertinent information regarding radionuclide therapy, including the identity and amount of radioactive material, date and time of administration, and the nature and projected duration of radiation precautions *shall* be included in the medical record. In addition, any measurements or calculations for determining the time post-administration at which the patient may be released from medical confinement and for post-release precautions *should* be included as part of the medical record.

2.2.3 *Dose Limits for Patients' Families and the Public*

The prospects of medical treatment, pain and suffering and even death of a family member create anxiety and stress within a family. At such times a family will tend to draw closer together to provide emotional and physical support to the patient. Family members often spend additional time with the patient, especially if treatment is palliative rather than curative. Measures to restrict access to a patient may be met with resistance by both patient and family, especially if they extend beyond a few days and are prescriptive, such as confinement in a medical facility. Access restrictions and confinement may heighten anxiety and stress of both patient and family. Accordingly, the ALARA principles outlined previously require that radiation protection standards applied to patients' families not be as restrictive as those standards for the public. This principle was first stated in NCRP Report No. 37 (NCRP, 1970) and is confirmed in this Report. Because radiation treatments are events that occur no more than a few times, or more likely once in the course of a lifetime, exposure of patients' families from radionuclide therapy *should* be considered as an "infrequent" exposure with an effective dose limit of 5 mSv (NCRP, 1993b). In addition, a member of a patient's family may be permitted to receive up to 50 mSv y^{-1} on the recommendation of the treating physician. When family members are likely to receive exposures >5 mSv annually, they *should* receive training and individual monitoring (NCRP, 1995b). The recommendation of the treating physicians *shall* be recorded in the patient record. Pregnant women and children *shall not* exceed 1 mSv y^{-1}.

For the purpose of applying radiation exposure limits, members of the public include other patients, visitors to the medical facility, such as family members of other patients in the facility, and staff who are not specifically trained in radiation safety. Other patients confined in the medical facility may be unintentionally exposed to patients receiving radionuclide therapy. The usual source of this exposure is occupancy of a room immediately adjacent to a patient receiving therapy. The effective doses to persons who have no familial connections to the patient and for whom there is no emotional benefit *shall* be limited to 1 mSv y^{-1}. Special considerations for women are included in Sections 3 and 4 of this Report and may be found in NCRP Commentary No. 9 (NCRP, 1994).

Some patients may be released while still containing measurable amounts of activity. Patients *should* be transported using a private car. Mass transit *should not* be used if an individual passenger or transit worker could receive >1 mSv annually. Coworkers who come into contact with a patient treated with radioactive sources *should not* receive an annual radiation dose >1 mSv. The doses to children or pregnant members of the family *shall not* exceed 1 mSv y^{-1}. Toward this end, facilities *should* ensure that family members clearly understand the appropriate precautions. Application of this limit is discussed further in Section 3 of this Report.

2.2.4 *Personal Monitoring and Bioassays*

Many aspects of this Report focus on the patient under treatment. However, there is also the potential for significant occupational doses to staff who treat or care for the patient. The monitoring of doses to radiation workers is the subject of NCRP Report No. 122 (NCRP, 1995b). For staff who do not prepare radiopharmaceutical or brachytherapy sources, a single dosimeter worn on the trunk is usually sufficient. Staff who prepare radiopharmaceutical or brachytherapy sources, especially those for therapy, usually use localized shielding to protect the trunk of the body. For those persons, monitoring of the dose to the extremities, forearms or other critical organs may require using additional dosimeters.

The RSO *shall* consider the specific personal monitoring needs of persons preparing therapeutic amounts of radiopharmaceuticals or sealed sources for use in brachytherapy. NCRP Report No. 122 provides additional guidance for this situation. The program *shall* provide authority to enforce the use of personal monitoring devices. The results of personal monitoring may require interpretation and *should* be left to the judgment of the RSO. Monitored staff *shall* be made aware of personal monitoring results at appropriate frequencies determined by the RSO, both as a safeguard for their own health and to provide an opportunity for the worker to make suggestions on maintaining doses ALARA.

Certain radiopharmaceutical therapies may require that staff prepare or use radioactive sources that have a volatile component. The classical example of this is the use of ^{131}I sodium iodide. In these cases, the RSO *shall* establish a bioassay program consistent with regulatory requirements and complexity of the program at the facility. The use of closed preparation systems and specific ion-exchange column preparations *shall* be considered to minimize the doses received by staff. The use or availability of properly ventilated hoods *shall* be part of an ALARA program for volatile materials. The design of an operational radiation safety program is discussed in NCRP Report No. 127 (NCRP, 1998).

2.3 Staffing

The staffing of medical facilities varies reflecting the patient load, the complexity of the practice, the research and education programs and, to some extent, the culture of the facility. The descriptions below are meant to provide a basis for considerations of the type of staffing necessary to conduct a program as well as to provide some guidance to management.

2.3.1 *Physician*

Radioactive sources *shall* be administered to patients by or under the supervision of a physician who possesses a license to practice medicine and who is qualified by appropriate training and experience. U.S. Nuclear Regulatory Commission (NRC) or Agreement States promulgate requirements that define the training and experience required for various categories of radioactive source administrations, both diagnostic and therapeutic. Physician specialists, such as ophthalmologists or cardiologists, may meet the requirements of various licensing subcategories as defined by the regulations. These specialists are usually restricted to a specific type of application, such as use of radioactive eye plaques or the placement of radioactive cardiac stents, respectively. For the purposes of this Report, the larger groupings of nuclear-medicine physicians or radiation oncologists are considered.

Typically, the nuclear-medicine physician and the radiation oncologist, by virtue of training and education, experience, and professional credentials, including certification and licensure, have the ultimate responsibility for the planning, delivery and follow-up of patients undergoing radiopharmaceutical therapy or brachytherapy. This responsibility includes the protection of the patient, facility personnel, visitors, and other individuals from unnecessary radiation exposure. Although consultation with referring physicians is necessary in the planning of such therapies, the nuclear-medicine physician or the radiation oncologist *shall* make the ultimate decisions regarding such therapies. In larger facilities, one or more of these specialists *should* serve on the Radiation Safety Committee (RSC) of the medical facility and provide consultation to the Committee as necessary. In facilities with emergency departments, the nuclear-medicine physician or radiation oncologist may also serve as the designated radiation emergency physician.

The responsibilities of the nuclear-medicine physician and the radiation oncologist include, in consultation with the RSO, the determination of whether medical confinement of patients for radiation protection is required. The formulation of radiation precautions for the staff of the medical facility and for visitors, as well as the formulation of and advice given to the patient and to members of the patient's family regarding post-release radiation precautions, including the duration of such precautions, is the responsibility of the RSO.

2.3.2 *Radiation Safety Officer*

In any medical facility in which radiation or radioactive sources are used a radiation safety officer (RSO) *shall* be designated who will have the responsibility to establish and the authority to enforce policies and procedures concerning safety and regulatory compliance in the use of radioactive sources (NCRP, 1998). Facility management *shall* empower the RSO with the necessary institutional authority to enforce such polices and procedures, including termination of the use of radioactive sources, and enable the RSO to have direct access to facility executive management. The training and experience of the RSO *shall* be commensurate with the complexity of the program and may be specified by a regulatory authority according to the type of licensure required by the program. These specifications may include certification by appropriate professional organizations (*e.g.*, American Board of Health Physics, American Board of Radiology, or American Board of Medical Physics).

Several states have enacted licensure laws that require that medical physicists be licensed. In some of these states, persons practicing the subspecialties of medical physics, including medical health physics, *shall* be specifically licensed. Licensure laws for medical physicists are pending in other states. Facilities in states with licensure laws *should* ensure that the physicists practicing in their facility are licensed or practicing under the supervision of a licensed physicist. In facilities with limited programs (*e.g.*, clinics limited to routine diagnostic uses of radiopharmaceuticals) it may be acceptable for a radiologist certified by the American Board of Radiology or a nuclear-medicine physician certified by the American Board of Nuclear Medicine to be appointed as the facility RSO.

Some of the duties of the RSO include:

- determination of radiation doses received by occupationally-exposed individuals and the public in and around the medical facility;

- promulgation of procedures for minimizing radiation exposure of such individuals;
- specification of precautions to be followed by patients treated with therapeutic amounts of radioactive sources;
- education and training of staff;
- education and training of the patient and the patient's family on post-release precautions;
- disposal of radioactive waste;
- removal of radioactive contamination;
- inventory and receipt of radioactive sources;
- consultation on shielding design;
- supervision of procedures that ensure the accuracy of the quantities of the administered radionuclides; and
- service on the RSC.

The RSO need not personally perform these duties and may delegate them to appropriately trained persons. However, when such delegations are made, the RSO *shall* be responsible for ensuring that the duties are performed correctly. Throughout this Report, any reference to the radiation safety officer (RSO), includes that individual and any authorized designees such as radiation safety staff.

2.3.3 *Medical Physicist and Nuclear Pharmacist*

For any program utilizing radioactive sources for therapeutic purposes, the services of a medical physicist *shall* be available on-site either on a full- or part-time basis. A qualified medical physicist *shall* be responsible for the supervision of the quality-control (QC) program in brachytherapy. For programs in nuclear medicine, a qualified medical physicist, a qualified nuclear pharmacist, or a nuclear-medicine physician *should* supervise the QC programs. For programs in nuclear medicine, the qualified nuclear pharmacist *should* perform a drug regimen review as required by state pharmacy regulations and the Joint Commission on Accreditation of Health Care Organizations. For facilities with programs in both nuclear medicine and brachytherapy, the services of medical physicists specializing in those areas will be necessary. The professional training and experience required of the medical physicist *shall* be commensurate with the complexity of the program and *should* include specialty board certification by appropriate professional organizations.

The duties of the medical physicist *should* include:

- calibration of equipment used for the assay of activity;
- calibration of brachytherapy sources;
- development of treatment plans;
- QC of nuclear-medicine imaging equipment;
- patient dosimetry;
- supervision of dosimetrists; and
- supervision of technologists.

The duties of a qualified nuclear pharmacist *should* include:

- assessing each patient's medication related needs;
- performing a patient drug regimen review prior to the therapeutic administration;
- procuring and dispensing of therapeutic radiopharmaceuticals;
- assaying the radioactive dosage;
- performing QC of the equipment used for the assay of activity;
- ensuring that the drug is of acceptable quality, purity and strength;
- ensuring that the radiopharmaceutical is compounded according to the specifications; established by the U.S. Pharmacopoeia (USP, 2004a);
- ensuring that the therapeutic radiopharmaceutical is prepared in the proper dosage form for the specific patient use (*e.g.*, capsule, injection, suspension or solution); and
- ensuring that considerations for pediatric dosing are reviewed and appropriate.

2.3.4 *Radiation Therapist and Nuclear-Medicine Technologist*

In many facilities using radioactive sources, there will usually be radiation therapists, formerly called radiation-therapy technologists, and nuclear-medicine technologists, the number of each will depend on the size of the program. These individuals will have undergone a period of training specified by professional registries or state licensing programs. Their responsibilities include assisting the radiation oncologist or nuclear-medicine physician in the delivery of the radioactive materials. The specific role of the radiation therapist in HDR remote afterloading is discussed in Section 4 and Appendix B. In nuclear-medicine applications, the technologist prepares the computerized data in a format suitable for interpretation by the nuclear-medicine physician. Depending on the program in specific facilities, nuclear-medicine technologists may also assist in the radiopharmacy and may dispense and may inject radiopharmaceuticals into patients.

2.3.5 *Dosimetrist*

Larger radiation-oncology programs employ the services of medical dosimetrists to assist the physician and medical physicist in the preparation and evaluation of treatment plans. These persons will have undergone a period of training under a qualified medical physicist and radiation oncologist and *should* have professional certification. The role of the dosimetrist in certain brachytherapy applications is discussed in Section 4 and Appendix B.

2.3.6 *Nurse*

Nurses who are specially trained in caring for patients treated with therapeutic amounts of radionuclides may be assigned to full- or part-time duty in nuclear medicine, radiation oncology, or a nursing unit that provides care for radionuclide therapy patients. These individuals *should* receive training by the authorized user and RSO that is more detailed than training provided to other nursing groups. Historically, nurses have played a variety of roles in these areas including the preparation of applicators and sealed sources for patient procedures in radiation oncology. In more recent times, the role of the nurse has evolved into a clinical support role for the radiation oncologist and nuclear medicine physician. The duties of the nurse may include evaluation of the mental and physical status of the patient, injection of diagnostic doses of radiopharmaceuticals, making the physician aware of unusual or aberrant symptoms or events, and assistance in patient emergencies.

2.3.7 *Physician-in-Training*

Some facilities may sponsor physician residency training programs. Larger facilities may also sponsor specialty fellowships in subspecialty areas such as brachytherapy. The physicians enrolled in these programs are licensed to practice medicine, and have elected to pursue a radiological specialty. Specialty certification boards require that these physicians acquire skills that will involve the administration of radioactive materials to patients. An experienced specialist physician *shall* supervise these physicians during their training period and *should* be on the premises during the administration of therapeutic quantities of radioactive materials to patients. The specialist physician or the RSO *shall* train fellows and residents in emergency procedures, regulatory requirements, and radiation safety procedures.

Teaching hospitals may provide opportunities for medical students to rotate through certain specialties or subspecialties, including the subspecialties of radiology. Although these students will not be involved in the administration of radioactive materials, they may be present when radioactive materials are administered. The role of these students and the requirements for supervision *shall* be clearly defined in the hospital procedure manuals. The requirements for monitoring *shall* be defined by the RSO as part of the radiation safety program.

2.4 Radiation Safety Committee

A medical-radiation facility, where therapeutic quantities of radionuclides are administered, *shall* have a standing radiation safety committee (RSC) that *shall* include at a minimum the RSO, a representative of management, a nurse and other individuals including physicians who have background and experience in radiation safety and the utilization of radiation and radioactive material. In large programs, the RSC *should* also include representatives with expertise in areas such as nuclear medicine, radiation oncology, nuclear pharmacy, radiation physics, and biomedical sciences. The RSC *shall* meet at regular intervals to review the routine and investigative uses of radioactive materials, to review the facility's radiation safety program, to review specific radiation safety questions or events, and to review institutional policy. The frequency of meetings required will depend on the complexity of the program. Special meetings *should* be convened as necessary by the Chair or at the request of the RSO and written minutes of all meetings *shall* be maintained. For certain medical-radiation facilities a RSC may not be necessary and may be replaced by knowledgeable professionals authorized by the management of the facility to develop and oversee its radiation safety program.

2.5 Management Commitment

Management *shall* be involved in the oversight of the QA and radiation safety programs of the facility. The involvement includes the allocation of resources adequate to meet the needs of the program and participation in the activities of the RSC. These allocations *should* be considered along with the requirements of regulatory authority. There *should* be direct communication between the RSO and facility management to promptly address the needs of the program. Facility management *shall* provide the RSO with sufficient resources, authority and autonomy to implement the radiation safety program.

The management of medical facilities and other installations in which ionizing radiation is employed *shall* have specific written policies and procedures for establishing and complying with dose-limiting standards (NCRP, 1998; NRC, 2005). These policies and procedures are usually derived from recommendations of advisory bodies such as NCRP or regulations promulgated by governmental agencies in the form of laws, codes and licensing guides. An important component of the radiation safety program of any such installation is a formal ALARA policy and procedure such as described in NCRP Report No. 107 (NCRP, 1990). It is not sufficient for a medical facility simply to maintain personal exposures below recommended or regulatory limits. A facility *shall* have a written, proactive policy and procedure to formally and practically maintain personal exposures ALARA. A medical facility performing radionuclide therapy *shall* be prepared to provide adequate resources, financial and otherwise, to comply with personal exposure limits and the ALARA principle.

2.6 Methods for Limiting Personal Exposure

Sections 3 and 4 discuss specific precautions to be taken during radiopharmaceutical therapy and brachytherapy. This Section outlines general precautions and provides an overview of radiation protection techniques. Methods for limiting personal exposure in radiation installations can be classified as either physical (or engineered) safeguards, including instrumentation, or as procedural controls (NCRP, 1998). Physical safeguards include all devices used to restrict access of staff and other individuals to radiation sources or to reduce radiation levels. Section 5 of this Report deals with facility design.

Procedural controls include instructions to and formal training of personnel regarding performance of their duties in a specific manner for the purpose of limiting radiation exposure. Details of such controls *should* be incorporated into institutional or departmental policies and procedures (NCRP, 1989; 1998). Regularly scheduled periodic radiation monitoring of occupationally-exposed personnel and in the work areas is necessary to ensure the adequacy of and compliance with physical safeguards and established procedural controls.

Procedures for handling radioactive materials *shall* conform to good radiation safety practice. Personnel working with unsealed radioactive sources *shall* wear disposable gloves and appropriate protective clothing, such as laboratory coats or disposable gowns. Personal dosimeters *shall* be worn when working with beta-, photon- and neutron-emitting radionuclides or in areas where radiation-producing equipment is present when potential doses warrant them. When working with large quantities of pure beta-emitting radionuclides, thermoluminescent dosimeters such as ring badges may be required. The necessity for monitoring and criteria for the monitoring program *shall* be part of the radiation safety program. To the extent possible, unsealed radioactive sources *should* be handled on plastic-backed absorbent pads and paper behind shielding as necessary. The amount and type of shielding necessary *should* be determined in consultation with the RSO. Eating, drinking, smoking, mouth pipetting, and other techniques that have the potential for accidental inhalation or ingestion of radioactive materials *shall* be forbidden in areas where radioactive materials are used. Applying cosmetics, handling contact lenses or other personal items have the potential to transfer radioactive materials to the exterior surface of the skin or other areas. These actions *shall* be forbidden in areas where radioactive materials are used. Laboratory coats and some form of eye protection (*e.g.*, safety glasses or splash guards) *shall* routinely be worn when handling radioactive materials in a pharmacy setting.

Radiopharmaceuticals and brachytherapy sources *shall* be transported in shielded containers if warranted by the amount of activity. The shielding of these containers *should* conform to the ALARA principles, and consultation with the RSO on appropriate shielding may be necessary. Protective equipment listed above and, including disposable gloves and shielded syringes *shall* be used during the administration of radiopharmaceuticals. The necessity of other protective equipment (*e.g.*, safety goggles, shoe covers) *should* be reviewed by the RSO. Impermeable absorbent materials such as plastic-backed absorbent pads *should* be placed underneath an injection or infusion site.

Consistent with patient safety and good quality medical care, personnel *should* spend as little time as necessary near or around radioactive material or patients treated with radiopharmaceuticals or brachytherapy sources, and *should* remain at distances as determined from exposure-rate measurements from such patients. Whenever practicable, in consultation with the RSO, portable shielding *should* be used to reduce further radiation levels to staff, especially during the hospitalization of radioactive patients.

2.7 Inventory, Receipt and Storage

If radioactive materials are packaged and shipped according to regulatory standards, the potential for inadvertent exposure is minimal. It is rare that a package is damaged during shipment sufficient to cause a radiation hazard. Packages containing radioactive sources *should* be delivered directly to the radiation safety office or to the brachytherapy or nuclear-medicine facility, received by an authorized individual in that facility and surveyed and secured upon arrival as outlined below.

In some instances delivery of radioactive sources may occur when the brachytherapy or nuclear-medicine facility is closed and there is no member of that facility available to receive the delivery. A written procedure approved by the facility's management *shall* be in place for off-hour deliveries. This procedure *should* include information for the facility's security or other approved personnel to gain access to the brachytherapy, nuclear medicine, or other appropriate secured area for receipt and storage of deliveries. Packages containing radioactive sources *shall not* be left unattended or unsecured.

Packages containing radioactive sources *shall* be examined and opened with the use of disposable gloves and other protective clothing. Packages *shall* be inspected immediately upon receipt for any sign of damage such as breakage, moisture or discoloration of the outer packing. As soon as possible after receipt, packages *shall* be monitored for external radiation levels using a radiation survey meter. Surface contamination *should* be determined by wipe testing. If the measured exposure rate is not consistent with the package label, if the removable surface contamination exceeds action levels established by the RSO, or if it appears that the package is damaged, the RSO or designee *shall* be contacted immediately. Once a package is opened, the inner container *should* be inspected for any breakage or leakage. The inner container *should* be wipe tested for contamination. The inner container label and the packing slip *should* be cross-checked to verify the vendor, the identity and physical and chemical forms of the radionuclide, the activity present, and date and time of calibration. Any deviations *shall* be discussed with the vendor and resolved before the material is used. These data *shall* be recorded in the facility's records. The packing material and empty packages *shall* be monitored for radioactive contamination using a survey meter before disposal. If radioactively contaminated, these materials *shall* be treated as radioactive waste. If free of contamination, the radiation/activity labels *shall* be removed or obliterated before disposal of the packaging as non-radioactive waste.

All vials or other vessels that contain radioactive materials *shall* be labeled with "caution radioactive material" labels. Such labels *shall* provide the identity of the radionuclide, physical or chemical forms of the radionuclide, activity, and date and time of calibration. Items that contain significant quantities of activity *shall* be stored in shielded containers, typically made of lead because the volumes are not large, with a thickness of shielding appropriate to the radionuclide and total activity present. Containers *should* be stored on plastic-backed absorbent pads, in shielded cabinets or drawers or behind lead or lead and low atomic-number combination shields (*e.g.*, lead acrylic). For certain radiopharmaceuticals that must be stored at low temperatures, a refrigerator may be lined with lead or a refrigerator may be located in an appropriately shielded area. Radioactive materials *shall* be stored in secured, controlled areas, such as a radiopharmacy or "hot lab," conspicuously posted with "caution radioactive material" warning signs. If personnel inside these areas could receive a dose of 0.05 mSv in any 1 h, the door *shall* be posted with a "caution radiation area" sign. These areas require appropriate security. A security expert *should* be consulted to ensure that security objectives are met. It may be advisable or necessary to require that persons entering these areas wear protective clothing such as a laboratory coat and a personal dosimeter for entry. All such controlled areas *shall* be regularly monitored for ambient radiation levels and radioactive contamination. Items such as food, beverages and medications *shall not* be stored in the same area as radioactive materials.

2.8 Surveys

The following sections outline some of the types of surveys that may be necessary in a program that utilizes therapeutic quantities of radioactive materials. These discussions are, of necessity, generic and *should* be supplemented with a specific program designed by the RSO.

2.8.1 *Ambient Exposure Rates*

A suitable radiation survey meter *shall* be available to measure ambient exposure or air kerma for calculation of absorbed dose or dose-equivalent rates. Such devices *shall* provide measurement in roentgen, rad, gray, rem or sievert per unit of time. The limits of measurement and characteristics of survey meters vary widely. It is critical to match the type of survey meter used with the characteristics of the radiation being measured. This will be particularly important in the measurement of low-energy radiations such as the emissions from ^{125}I and radionuclides with similar energies. The most common types of devices for measurement of exposure rate are the Geiger-Mueller (GM) counter and the ion chamber (St. Germain, 1995). The limitations of pulse-rate detectors in the measurement of exposure rates *should* be understood by the person performing the survey. Scintillation probes are high-sensitivity solid-state detectors. The sensitivity of the crystal will be specified for a range of photon energies. These detectors may be particularly useful for monitoring of low-energy photons with energies <60 keV. The ionization chamber, GM counter, scintillation probe with thin entrance windows, or other radiation detection instrument *should* be calibrated to provide readings in appropriate units if measurements of exposure, absorbed dose, or dose equivalent are to be performed. Because of the limited penetration of beta particles and other particulate radiations, the ability of each type of survey meter to detect these radiations *should* be clearly understood. The use of beta shields or caps may allow for measurements in fields of mixed radiations. Survey meters *should* include a "battery check" function. Survey meters *should* be checked for proper functional operation immediately prior to use with a low activity "check source," which can be an integral part of the instrument. These devices *shall* be calibrated at least annually and records of the calibrations *shall* be maintained. Performance standards for radiation surveys can be found in the recommendations of the American National Standards Institute (ANSI, 2001).

Properly calibrated ionization chambers, GM counters, and other survey meters can measure exposure rates at a point in air. Conversion of these measurements to absorbed dose and dose equivalent requires several calculational steps. However, for photons <1 MeV, absorbed dose and dose equivalent are approximately equal to measured exposures at the corresponding point in air (Appendix A.1). For beta particles with energies <3 MeV, the absorbed dose and dose-equivalent rates to skin may be similarly equated with the measured exposure rate at the corresponding point in air. These simplifying assumptions are conservatively safe, and overestimate the actual absorbed dose and dose equivalent corresponding to a measured exposure rate in air because the substantial reduction achieved by an irradiated individual's body is ignored.

2.8.2 *Removable Contamination (Wipe Tests)*

Radioactive contamination in the work environment that is removable can deposit on the skin or enter the body and irradiate an individual internally. Therefore, assay of removable radioactive contamination on all potentially contaminated surfaces and on sealed radioactive sources *shall* be performed at regular intervals and whenever contamination is suspected. Nonremovable radioactive contamination (*i.e.*, fixed contamination) contributes only to external exposure and its contribution is incorporated in the determination of ambient exposure rate. Assay of removable radioactive contamination is typically performed using a "wipe test." In such a test, a representative area of ~100 cm² of a potentially contaminated surface is wiped with a dry or wet material (*e.g.*, filter paper) and the wipe is counted in a counting system appropriate to the radioactive materials being used (*e.g.*, a liquid scintillation counter). The choice of which wipe material to use, the presence or absence of water or any solvent on a wipe *should* be discussed with the RSO to optimize the information obtained. The resulting gross count rates are converted to net count rates by subtracting a background, or blank, count rate. Net count rates are converted to activity by adjusting the count rate by the system counting efficiency for the radionuclide in question. Results *shall* be recorded and archived. Records *shall* be maintained for periods established by regulatory agencies or for periods established by the facility, whichever is longer (NCRP, 1992a).

Surfaces notably susceptible to radioactive contamination include doorknobs, drawer handles, light switches, toilet seats and bathroom fixtures in patient rooms, telephones and telephone mouthpieces used by patients, and computer keyboards. If removable contamination is detected by wipe testing, the contaminated surface(s) *shall* be decontaminated by appropriate techniques. The decontamination techniques *should* minimize the spread of contamination over a larger area. Any radioactively contaminated disposable items (*e.g.*, gloves and paper toweling) *shall* be held for decay in storage or otherwise disposed of as radioactive waste. Following decontamination, the contaminated area *should* be wipe tested again and, if detectable removable contamination is still present, decontamination *should* be repeated until levels approaching background are attained. However, the RSO can establish institutional levels of removable contamination below which no further decontamination is required.

2.8.3 *Airborne Activity*

The most common source of airborne activity in medical practice is the use of any of the radioisotopes of iodine (*e.g.*, ^{125}I or ^{131}I). Volatilization is most likely to occur when sealed vials of acidic solutions containing radioiodide (sodium iodide) are first opened and when peptides or proteins, including antibodies, are radioiodinated. Radioiodinations *shall* be performed in closed systems or in a fume hood equipped with an iodine-trapping filter, such as an activated charcoal filter. The exhaust *shall* be vented to a suitable exhaust stack approved for this purpose by the RSO. The filter *shall* be replaced according to the manufacturer's recommended schedule or when the pressure gradient across the filter falls below an acceptable level. The flow rate through the fume hood *shall* be measured at least annually. In large programs evaluation of radioactive releases *shall* be performed at least annually. Real-time stack monitoring *should* be performed in systems such as medical cyclotrons used for production of short-lived radionuclides. The design of such systems *should* be reviewed by an expert in air monitoring systems.

Measurement of radioactive contamination in air can be performed by drawing air through a suitable filter using a vacuum pump and measuring the activity retained on the filter. An air pump capable of pumping from 10 to 40 ft^3 min^{-1} and sampling times from 5 min to 2 h *should* be used to obtain a reasonable sample in a short time. A calibrated flow meter is required to measure the volume of air pumped per unit time.

2.9 Personal Monitoring

2.9.1 *External Monitoring*

Personal monitoring for external exposure *shall* be performed for all occupationally-exposed individuals who, in the judgment of the RSO, have the potential to receive >10 % of the annual effective dose limit during the normal course of their duties and individuals who enter high radiation areas. Facilities *shall* use personal radiation dosimeters from vendors that are accredited by the National Voluntary Laboratory Accreditation Program. Extremity dosimeters *shall* be worn when an individual's extremities are expected to be closer to the source than the body and could likely exceed 10 % of the dose limit.

2.9.2 *Bioassay*

The term bioassay refers to the radiological analysis of:

- the entire body in a whole-body radiation-detection system;
- a portion of the body using an external collimated radiation detector to determine activity content in a specific area or organ (*e.g.*, the thyroid);

- body fluids (*e.g.*, saliva, sputum, blood);
- excreta (*e.g.*, urine, feces, exhaled breath, or perspiration); and
- tissue samples (*e.g.*, hair, fingernail parings).

Bioassay is used to determine the activity present in an individual. The optimal type of bioassay procedure to use depends on the chemical and physical form of the radioactive material, the radiation emissions, mode of entry of activity into the body, and the characteristic biodistribution and effective half-lives *in vivo*. Performance criteria for radiobioassays including statistical testing, reporting of results and record retention have been established by ANSI (1996). By application of appropriate biological models and kinetic parameters, bioassay measurements are converted to body or organ activity burdens and, ultimately, to estimates of absorbed dose. Whether inhaled, ingested, absorbed through intact skin or passed through breaks in the skin, soluble radioactive materials will be transferred over time to excreta, particularly urine. This process will rely on blood transport and can be detected and measured by radioassay *ex vivo* of urine or blood samples in a scintillation well counter or liquid scintillation counter.

Internal radioactive contamination from photon emitters may be detected and measured by total or partial body counting using a variety of organ uptake probes. Unless internal radioactive contamination is substantial, a gamma camera may not have sufficient sensitivity for bioassays. Removing the collimator and using the gamma camera in a counting (*i.e.*, nonimaging) mode may provide adequate sensitivity if the background counting rate is not excessively high. High resolution gamma-ray spectrometers may be useful if the identity of the radionuclide is in question.

In radiopharmaceutical therapy, possible internal contamination can occur from ingestion of liquids or contact of a radiolabeled compound with bare skin. In a rare circumstance, an individual may accidentally inject a portion of a compound into his own body while preparing the radiopharmaceutical. Reporting requirements for accidental exposures and procedures for bioassay and estimates of any dose received *should* be a part of the institution's policy and procedure manual.

During the radiochemical labeling of compounds with ^{131}I or ^{125}I, significant intakes can occur due to the oxidation of radioactive iodine and the volatilization and inhalation of the radioiodine as a gas (I_2). The rapid uptake and long retention of radioiodine by the thyroid requires a sensitive bioassay of internal radioiodine contamination. Thyroid burden *should* be measured using a thyroid uptake probe. Personnel who prepare or administer therapeutic amounts of radioiodine as well as personnel who radiolabel peptides and proteins with significant amounts of radioiodine *should* be monitored as part of an established thyroid bioassay program. There may be regulatory requirements for a thyroid bioassay program and the RSO *should* advise on these requirements. For nuclear-medicine personnel involved in therapeutic procedures, these assays *should* take place typically within 1 to 3 d after the administration.

2.10 Radioactive Waste Disposal

Radiopharmaceutical therapy generates low-level radioactive waste, mostly in the form of dry waste, including empty vials, syringes, intravenous tubing, disposable gloves, absorbent pads, paper toweling, gauze, contaminated disposable eating utensils, and partially decayed radioactive fiducial markers and calibration sources. Brachytherapy procedures may generate small amounts of radioactive waste, however these wastes may be longer-lived than radiopharmaceutical wastes (*e.g.*, spent ^{125}I seeds). Depending on the volume of radioactive waste generated and the medical facility's capacity for waste storage, disposal may be accomplished by one of the methods described in the following subsections.

2.10.1 *Return to Vendor*

Partially decayed radioactive fiducial markers and standard calibration sources, especially larger sources, *should* be returned to the vendor for disposal. Some vendors will accept seeds containing radioactive materials that were intended for use in brachytherapy procedures but were not used. Whenever possible, seeds *should* be returned to the vendor. However, when this is not possible, seeds will have to be held for decay or disposed as low-level radioactive waste. Commercial radiopharmacies will often accept their unit-dose syringes and unit- and multi-dose vials used for therapeutic radiopharmaceuticals. Vendor acceptance of such items *should* be confirmed explicitly before purchase and any disposal costs specified at the time of purchase, because vendors may not otherwise accept them.

2.10.2 *Storage for Radioactive Decay*

Radionuclides that will decay to background levels within a reasonably short period of time (*e.g.*, several months to a few years) may be stored for decay. The volume of radioactive waste that can be stored on-site will depend on storage capacity within the facility. Such locations *should* be in a low-occupancy, secure, and posted area of the facility and adequately shielded as required. Prior to disposal or recycling of decayed radioactive waste, such materials *shall* be monitored with a suitable survey meter in a low background area to verify that the activity is acceptably low or not detectable, and all "radioactive material" labeling *shall* be removed or obliterated prior to disposal or recycling. Disposal or recycling of these materials must meet applicable regulatory requirements. The RSO *should* be consulted regarding any disposal requirements. Lead containers used for storage or shipment of radioactive materials *should* be surveyed by wipe testing and with a survey meter to verify the absence of removable activity and recycled according to applicable environmental regulations.

2.10.3 *Transfer to a Radioactive Waste Facility or Broker*

Radioactive waste that cannot be returned to the vendor or that has a physical half-life beyond that which practically allows on-site decay in storage may be transferred to a licensed commercial facility or broker. The identity, amount and chemical/physical form of the radionuclide(s) *shall* be specified on the shipping manifest, and packaging and transport regulations *shall* be understood by the licensed shipper. The regulations for shipping and transport are complex and may also require an understanding of the chemical or biological hazard in the waste as well as the activity. Transport of radioactive waste in interstate commerce is governed by the regulations of the U.S. Department of Transportation, NRC, and other agencies claiming jurisdiction (DOT, 2006). It is, therefore, important that the person preparing wastes for shipment be familiar with these regulations by receiving training in these areas. The ultimate disposal of these materials will rely on techniques employed at the disposal site. Volume reduction (*e.g.*, supercompaction or incineration) *should* be considered to reduce the overall volume of the waste.

2.10.4 *Disposal via Sanitary Sewer*

Excreta (including excreta collected in urine bags and bedpans) from patients who were administered radiopharmaceuticals *should* be discharged through the sanitary sewer. After disposal of liquid patient waste in this manner, the toilet *should* be flushed several times and the surfaces rinsed thoroughly with a gentle stream of water to avoid aerosolization or splashing of radioactively contaminated liquid. Disposal of other forms of radioactive liquid waste (*e.g.*, from laboratories that do not generate chemical hazards or biological waste) *should* rely on sufficient dilution of the waste at the point of disposal and *shall* be documented and recorded as part of the institution's overall program. The RSO *shall* ensure that liquid radioactive waste, excluding patient excreta, discharged into the sewer does not exceed regulatory limits and *shall* record each disposal.

2.11 Training

Training is an essential component of the radiation safety program in a medical-radiation facility. Well-trained staff are essential in implementing the radiation safety program and in presenting a positive, competent image to patients. All employees, including technical, clinical nursing, and support personnel, involved with patients who contain radioactive materials *shall* attend a facility-specific radiation safety program or complete equivalent online training. The exact content of this training *should* be tailored by the RSO to the level of involvement of the staff and their potential for radiation exposure. Training of such personnel *should* occur as soon as possible after new employees begin work. Refresher training *should* be provided annually, or whenever there are significant modifications of an operational procedure that may, in the judgment of the RSO, affect radiation exposure to employees or members of the public. Training content *should* include the nature of activity, the medical uses of radiation and radioactive materials, limitations on exposure time and proximity to radiation sources, use and the limitations of physical safeguards, waste handling procedures, applicable regulatory requirements, prohibited activities and other procedural controls and emergency procedures (NCRP, 1989; 2000). Training content *should* emphasize practical issues that affect radiation exposure and *should* be tailored to the specific tasks performed by personnel. A description of the training material and documentation of completion of training *shall* be retained. Whenever possible, didactic training *should* be supplemented by supervised practical training (*i.e.*, on-the-job training) specific to the tasks performed by the person being trained.

2.12 Record Keeping

Documentation provides evidence of the reliability and effectiveness of a radiation safety program. Records *shall* be maintained for periods established by regulatory agencies or for periods established by the facility, whichever is longer (NCRP, 1992b; 1995b; 1998). Among the records that *should* be maintained as part of the overall program are:

- radioactive materials receipt, inventory, distribution and disposal, including radiopharmaceutical prescriptions and brachytherapy written directives;
- radiation survey data, including measurements of ambient radiation levels and surface radioactive contamination including facility diagrams indicating the sites of such measurements;
- airborne activity data;
- radioactive effluent data;
- monitoring records for all occupationally-exposed personnel, including bioassay data as appropriate;
- written policies and procedures for the radiation safety program;
- radiation safety training program, including the curriculum or lesson plans and attendance lists;
- RSC membership and minutes; and
- reports of unusual, radiologically significant occurrences and operational failures.

2.13 Transport of Patients and Patient Specimens

The movement within a facility of patients treated with diagnostic levels of radiopharmaceuticals or specimens from such patients represents a minimal level of radiation exposure for employees, patients, and members of the public. However, therapeutic quantities of radioactive materials in patients may cause increased exposure. Radiation doses will be a function of the activity remaining in the patient, the type and energy of the emitted radiation, the distribution of the radioactive material within the patient's body, the distance from the patient, the time spent in the vicinity of the patient and, in the case of certain radionuclides, the size (thickness) of the patient. When it is deemed necessary to administer radionuclide therapy on an inpatient basis, therapeutic quantities of radioactive materials *should* be administered in the patient's room to minimize the need for transportation of a radioactive patient. Once the therapeutic activity is administered, the patient *shall* remain in the hospital room except in emergencies (*e.g.*, the need for surgical intervention). The advice of the RSO *should* be sought for any special precautions (Section 6).

Specimens from patients treated with temporary implants of sealed radioactive sources (*e.g.*, patients with temporary gynecological implants) are not radioactive and may be transported without regard to activity. Urine specimens from patients treated with permanent implants (*e.g.*, ^{125}I seeds for prostate implants) may occasionally contain a seed. These specimens *should* be checked for the presence of a seed before being sent to the appropriate laboratory. Specimens from patients treated with radiopharmaceutical therapy may contain activity. It is usually not necessary to shield these specimens except when a large number of such specimens are stored in one location. In most cases, standard precautions will suffice for the handling of these specimens. The RSO *should* be consulted any time there are questions.

3. Radiopharmaceutical Therapy

Radiopharmaceutical therapy is the administration of unsealed radioactive material designed to elicit a therapeutic response as a result of internal irradiation of a target tissue. Therapeutic radiopharmaceuticals may be structurally simple (*e.g.*, ions) or complex materials into which the radioactive material has been incorporated (*e.g.*, monoclonal antibodies). Such radiopharmaceutical formulations may be solutions or colloidal suspensions with administration either systemic or local.

Historically, radioiodine (^{131}I) therapy of thyroid disease, including hyperthyroidism as well as localized and metastatic thyroid cancer, has been the most studied and successful application of radiopharmaceutical therapy. This success has largely resulted from the high and rapid uptake and long retention of iodide in thyroidal tissue, and little uptake in extra-thyroidal tissues. Although ^{131}I therapy of thyroid disease remains the most widely used form of radionuclide therapy, there are a number of newer and less frequently applied radionuclide therapies (Cheung *et al.*, 2001; Freeman and Blaufox, 1989; 1992; Harbert, 1987; Kramer and Cheung, 2001; Lashford *et al.*, 1988; Spencer, 1978).

Systemic therapies include:

- targeted radioimmunotherapy of cancer, particularly of leukemias and lymphomas;
- ^{32}P therapy of myeloproliferative diseases, especially *polycythemia vera*;
- meta-^{131}I-iodobenzylguanidine therapy of neuroendocrine cancers including pheochromocytomas and neuroblastomas; and
- palliation of bone pain secondary to skeletal metastases using bone-seeking radiopharmaceuticals such as ^{32}P, ^{89}Sr, ^{90}Y, ^{186}Re and ^{188}Re, hydroxyethylidene diphosphonate, ^{153}Sm ethylenediamene tetramethylene phosphonate, ^{117m}Sn, and diethylene triamine pentaacetic acid (DTPA).

Local/regional therapies include:

- intracavitary radioimmunotherapy and radiocolloid therapy of malignant effusions and ascites using beta emitters such as ^{32}P;
- intra-cystic radiocolloid therapy, principally using ^{32}P-chromic phosphate (*e.g.*, cystic intracranial tumors);
- intrathecal radioimmunotherapy and radiocolloid therapy of leptomeningeal tumors (*e.g.*, ^{131}I-labeled 3F8 monoclonal antibody);
- intra-articular radiocolloid therapy, also known as radiation synovectomy, synoviorthesis, or synoviolysis, of benign joint disease using ^{51}Cr, ^{186}Re, ^{90}Y as citrate or silicate, ^{153}Sm-hydroxyapatite, and ^{169}Er citrate; and
- intracranial infusion of labeled materials to treat residual disease following removal of the primary brain tumor (*e.g.*, ^{125}I labeled organic compounds for treatment of glioblastoma multiforme).

3.1 Systemic and Regional Therapies

In systemic therapy, a therapeutic radiopharmaceutical is administered either orally or parenterally, typically intravenously, for distribution throughout the patient's entire body *via* circulatory, secretory, metabolic and excretory processes. In this way, some activity is deposited in all tissues of the body. Each tissue irradiates and is irradiated by all other tissues of the body. Significant amounts of activity may be found in all bodily fluids such as blood, saliva, cerebrospinal fluid, and breast milk as well as in excreta (*e.g.*, feces, urine, perspiration and breath). In general, blood and urine contain the larger amounts of activity, especially in the first several days following administration. Also, radioactive small molecules (*i.e.*, molecular weight <50,000 dalton) that are not localized in target tissues will be rapidly excreted by the kidneys. However, some renal or hepatic localization may occur as a result of metabolism or transchelation. Large molecules, such as radiolabeled proteins and antibodies, are more pharmacokinetically complex. Although small polar metal chelates typically result in low hepatic uptake and biliary excretion, protein-bound chelates may enter hepatocytes and be catabolized to small molecules that subsequently may be excreted into the intestines or partially retained. In systemic therapy with photon-emitting radionuclides, there exists a significant radioactive contamination hazard from the radioactive excretions as well as an external irradiation hazard to individuals in the vicinity of the patient.

In regional therapy, the therapeutic radiopharmaceutical is introduced directly into a specific volume of the body, such as the pleural cavity, to mechanically deposit activity into the volume or on the surface of target organs. In this way, specificity of treatment is maximized. If little or no leakage of the radiopharmaceutical from the target tissue volume occurs, there is little or no activity in body fluids or excreta and, therefore, no significant contamination hazard. In the absence of significant biological clearance, the only means of elimination of activity is physical decay *in situ*. Therefore, the external irradiation hazard in regional therapy can persist longer than in systemic therapy.

With the continued development of new radiopharmaceuticals, management of patients who have received therapeutic amounts of radionuclides is becoming increasingly important and complex. A compilation of the properties of photon- and beta-emitting radionuclides commonly used in therapeutic radiopharmaceuticals is presented in Table 3.1.

3.2 Choice of Radionuclides

Selection of the optimal radionuclide is clearly critical to successful therapy. While it is difficult to generalize, dosimetric considerations can provide guidelines for the selection of appropriate therapeutic radionuclides (Hosain and Hosain, 1978; Spencer, 1978; Wessels and Rogus, 1984; Zanzonico *et al.*, 1995). If possible, the physical half-life of the radionuclide *should* be substantially longer than the uptake half-time and substantially shorter than the clearance half-time of the radiopharmaceutical in the target tissue. In this way, the amount of time the activity remains in the tissue and, therefore, the absorbed dose to the target tissue will be maximized while the dose to nontarget tissues will be minimized. In regional therapy, these considerations will not apply. Radiobiological considerations suggest that therapeutic radionuclides with excessively long physical half-lives may be undesirable (Ling, 1992). In practice, however, long-lived radionuclides may prove to be therapeutically effective.

Because self-irradiation (*i.e.*, dose from activity in the target tissue) generally represents the largest component of total absorbed dose in a target region, a therapeutic radionuclide should emit principally nonpenetrating (beta, alpha) radiation and little or no photon (x or gamma ray) radiation. To a first-order approximation, this corresponds to maximizing the ratio of the nonpenetrating to photon equilibrium dose constants. The nonpenetrating radiation

TABLE 3.1—Physical properties of photon- and beta-emitting radionuclides commonly used in therapeutic radiopharmaceuticals.

Radionuclide	Physical Half-Life	Specific Gamma-Ray Constant[a,b] ($R\ cm^2\ mCi^{-1}\ h^{-1}$)	Maximum Beta-Ray Energy (MeV)	Specific Bremsstrahlung Constant[a,b] ($R\ cm^2\ mCi^{-1}\ h^{-1}$)	
				Soft Tissue $Z_{eff} = 7.9$	Bone (calcium) $Z_{eff} = 21$
Photon- and Beta-Emitters					
^{131}I	8.04 d	2.23	0.81	0.000768	0.00204
^{177}Lu	6.7 d	0.222	0.497, 0.44	0.000385	0.00102
^{153}Sm	47 h	0.712	0.8	0.000597	0.00159
^{186}Re	89 h	0.143	1.07	0.00121	0.00322
^{188}Re	17 h	0.320	2.12	0.00154	0.00409
Beta-Emitters					
^{32}P	14.3 d	—	1.71	0.00405	0.0108
^{33}P	25.4 d	—	0.25	0.000658	0.00175
^{89}Sr [c]	50.5 h	—	1.49	0.00314	0.00843
^{90}Y	64.1 h	—	2.28	0.00564	0.015

[a]Values for constants from NUREG-1556, Vol. 9 (NRC, 2005), and, for ^{177}Lu only (Unger and Trubey, 1982).

[b]The specific gamma-ray constant is a physical quantity that is expressed in conventional units of $R\ cm^2\ mCi^{-1}\ h^{-1}$. The specific gamma-ray constant and the analogous specific bremsstrahlung are, therefore, expressed in these conventional units.

[c]Although ^{89}Sr emits a gamma ray, it is grouped with the beta emitters because the frequency of its gamma-ray emissions, <0.01 % per decay, is negligibly low.

must nonetheless be sufficiently energetic to actually irradiate target cell nuclei, the critical radiobiologic target within the cell (Warters et al., 1977). It is often desirable in practice that a radionuclide either itself emit photons in sufficient abundance and of suitable energy for external imaging or have an isotope that emits such radiations. For example, [85]Sr, which emits a 514 keV gamma ray, may be used as an imaging surrogate of the pure beta-emitter [89]Sr (Footnote c in Table 3.1), a radionuclide of strontium used therapeutically (Blake et al., 1988; Breen et al., 1992). Other radionuclides emit only high-energy beta particles ($e.g.$, ^{32}P with average energy 0.70 MeV) and there are no photon-emitting radionuclides of suitable half-life for quantitative imaging measurements. Nonetheless, the high-energy ^{32}P beta particle will undergo ~2 % bremsstrahlung energy-loss interactions in water or soft tissue and, like other radionuclides that emit high-energy beta particles such as the various radionuclides of yttrium, the resulting radiation can be scintigraphically counted and imaged (Balachandran et al., 1985; Boye et al., 1984; Feitelberg and Loevinger, 1955; Kaplan et al., 1981).

Alternatively for beta-emitting radionuclides for which a suitable photon-emitting radionuclide does not exist, chemical homologs of the therapeutic radiopharmaceutical labeled with a photon-emitting radionuclide may be used. For example, [111]In- and ^{90}Y-ibritumomab tiuxetan (an IgG$_1$ murine monoclonal antibody directed against the CD20 antigen found on the surface of normal and malignant B lymphocytes) are components of the Zevalin® (ibritumomab tiuxetan) (Biogen Idec, Cambridge, Massachusetts) regimen (Conti et al., 2005). Zevalin® is used for treatment of patients with relapsed or refractory low-grade, follicular, or transformed B-cell non-Hodgkin's lymphoma, and also for patients with follicular B-cell non-Hodgkin's lymphoma that is refractory to Rituxan® (rituximab) (Biogen Idec, Cambridge, Massachusetts) therapy. Yttrium-90-ibritumomab tiuxetan is the actual therapeutic component of the regimen but is labeled with the pure beta-emitter ^{90}Y and is not imageable. Photon-emitting ^{111}In-ibritumomab tiuxetan is, therefore, used as an imaging surrogate to verify, in advance of the therapeutic administration of ^{90}Y-ibritumomab tiuxetan, that the expected distribution of the labeled antibody is obtained.

The use of beta-emitting radionuclides simplifies certain radiation safety issues in radionuclide therapy. For beta energies <1 MeV used in such therapy, electrons have maximum ranges in water or soft tissue of only several millimeters and, thus, would be almost completely absorbed by the patient's tissues, effectively eliminating any external radiation hazard. However, a small portion of the beta-particle energy will be lost as bremsstrahlung resulting in the emission of generally low-energy photon radiation. As an example, for ^{32}P, the beta particle will undergo ~2 % bremsstrahlung energy loss yielding a photon energy spectrum with a broad maximum of ~70 keV (Balanchandran *et al.*, 1985). In practice, with the relatively low electron energies encountered in radionuclide therapy, the low abundance and energy of associated bremsstrahlung makes the external radiation hazard insignificant. Accordingly, there is no need to isolate or otherwise limit access to patients who have received radiopharmaceutical therapy with a beta emitter unless contamination is suspected (Zanzonico *et al.*, 1999). Standard precautions should be adequate for such patients. A list of liquid radioactive materials commonly used for therapeutic treatments is given in Table 3.2.

The use of radiopharmaceuticals labeled with alpha emitters is an emerging modality (McDevitt *et al.*, 1998; 1999; Sgouros, 1999). The use of these sources labeled to monoclonal antibodies offers the opportunity to deliver large doses of radiation with little or no external radiation hazard to staff taking care of these patients. Accordingly, there is no need to isolate or otherwise limit access to patients who have received radiopharmaceutical therapy with a alpha emitter unless contamination is anticipated. A listing of alpha-emitting radionuclides currently in use or under development for use with various compounds is given in Table 3.3.

Besides the foregoing dosimetric considerations, the selection of a therapeutic radionuclide depends on several circumstances including its availability, the cost of the radionuclide and the regulatory approval of the radiopharmaceutical.

3.3 Clinical Aspects

This Section discusses in generic terms equipment and procedures necessary to satisfy the clinical requirements for a radiopharmaceutical therapy program. This listing cannot be comprehensive and deals primarily with radiopharmaceuticals for which FDA has approved a new drug application, although research materials in investigational new drug application Phase II and III trials may be included. A listing of radionuclides and compounds commonly used for radiopharmaceutical therapy is given in Tables 3.1 and 3.2. This Section is intended to indicate requirements that may be incorporated into the larger clinical program within a medical facility.

TABLE 3.2—*Liquid radioactive materials commonly used for therapeutic treatment.*[a]

Radionuclide	Typical Activities Used[b]	Medical Use (chemical form)
[32]P	111 – 185 MBq	Polycythemia vera (sodium phosphate)
		Essential thrombocytosis (sodium phosphate)
		Synovectomy (chromic phosphate)
	296 – 444 MBq	Bone pain (sodium phosphate)
	370 – 555 MBq	Malignant effusions (chromic phosphate)
[131]I	185 – 740 MBq	Hyperthyroidism (sodium iodide)
	2.59 – 3.7 GBq	Thyroid ablation (sodium iodide)
	1.11 – 14.8 GBq	Thyroid cancer (sodium iodide)
	Activity required to deliver 65 – 75 Gy[c]	Lymphoma therapy (labeled antibody Tositumomab)
[89]Sr	148 MBq	Bone pain (strontium chloride)
[153]Sm	37 MBq kg^{-1} of body weight	Bone pain (samarium lexidronam, a chelate)
[90]Y	11.1 – 14.8 MBq kg^{-1} of body weight up to 1.19 GBq	Lymphoma therapy (yttrium-labeled antibody, ibritumomab tiuxetan)

[a]The actual activities used for any individual patient will be individually prescribed by the treating nuclear-medicine physician and may vary considerably from the amounts shown.

[b]The activities listed are only an indication of what may be used. This list is not a substitute for an individual prescription and is not a prescribing manual.

[c]The dose shown is an estimated whole-body absorbed dose. The prescribed activity will require a dose calculation prior to therapeutic administration. This compound is a monoclonal antibody.

TABLE 3.3—*Physical properties of alpha-emitting radionuclides currently in use or under development with various compounds.*

Radionuclide	Physical Half-Life	Energy (MeV)
^{225}Ac	10 d	5.9
^{211}At	7.2 h	5.8
^{212}Bi [a]	1.0 h	6.0
^{213}Bi [b]	46 min	5.8
^{224}Ra	3.71 d	5.7

[a]Generator-produced isotope; parent radionuclide is ^{224}Ra.
[b]Generator-produced isotope; parent radionuclide is ^{225}Ac.

3.3.1 *Instrumentation*

A medical facility performing radionuclide therapy *should* have instrumentation for measuring activity *in vivo* for the procedures performed. Some therapeutic administrations (*e.g.*, ^{89}Sr therapies) are performed with standard activities which are not customized to the individual patient, and assessment of the activity distribution may not be performed after the treatment. Typical instrumentation may include an uptake probe and one or more gamma cameras, preferably one of which has the capability of performing single-photon emission computed tomography imaging. Such instrumentation *should* be used to verify, at least qualitatively, the distribution of therapeutic radiopharmaceuticals in individual patients and, possibly, to quantify tissue activities for radiation dosimetry and treatment planning. However, with the use of beta-emitting radionuclides, including ^{32}P, ^{89}Sr, and ^{90}Y, imaging may be limited. The use of "imageable" surrogate radiopharmaceuticals for therapeutic agents labeled with such radionuclides may be necessary as discussed in the previous section.

Measurement of activity *in vivo* may be accomplished using a nonimaging gamma counting system consisting of a sodium-iodide [NaI (Tl)] detector generally used for ^{131}I thyroid uptake measurements. Modern, commercially available uptake probes are generally supplied as integrated, computerized systems with automated data acquisition and processing capabilities that yield results directly in terms of percent uptake of the administered activity.

Patient data are normalized by comparing the net count rates (*i.e.*, background corrected count rates) between that of a calibrated standard and the administered activity. As with all clinical instrumentation, a documented QA program for uptake probes *shall* be implemented. The program *should* include daily examination of pulse-height spectra to verify that the radionuclide-specific photopeaks are symmetric and centered within the corresponding photopeak energy windows. Daily measurement of counting efficiency and stability (net count rate per unit activity) *shall* be made using an independently calibrated standard traceable to the National Institute of Standards and Technology (NIST) to verify constancy over time, with or without other testing. Measurement of activity, typically prior to administration, can be accomplished using a dose calibrator (see Section 3.3.3 for a discussion of this instrument).

Radionuclides *in vivo* are most commonly measured using a gamma camera, also known as an Anger or scintillation camera, consisting of an energy-appropriate multihole collimator, a large-area "thin" sodium-iodide [Nal (Tl)] scintillation crystal, an array of up to 100 photomultiplier tubes, a high-voltage power supply, preamplifiers, amplifiers, analog or digital position and energy determination circuitry, energy discriminator, display, patient table/palette, and an electronic gantry. Modern, commercially available gamma cameras are supplied as integrated, computerized systems with automated data acquisition, processing, storage and display capabilities, associated software and online spatial linearity, energy and sensitivity corrections which may be updated to maintain optimum system performance. A documented QA program for gamma cameras *shall* be implemented, that includes daily examination of pulse height spectra, daily qualitative or quantitative evaluation of intrinsic or extrinsic uniformity, and weekly qualitative evaluation of intrinsic or extrinsic spatial resolution. A complete discussion of QA programs cannot be presented in this Report. However, information on such programs is available from the following organizations directly or from their websites: American College of Radiology, Society of Nuclear Medicine, the American Association of Physicists in Medicine, and the American Society of Nuclear Cardiology.

Instrumentation, typically a scintillation well counter system, *should* also be available to measure activity in patient samples, such as blood or urine. Additional instrumentation such as multichannel analyzers or radionuclide thin-layer-chromatography analyzers may be available as needed for testing of radionuclide purity or radiopharmaceutical assays.

3.3.2 *Prescription of Administered Activity*

There is currently no standardized algorithm for prescribing the administered activity in radionuclide therapy. Although an in-depth discussion is beyond the scope of this Report, a brief survey of such algorithms may be helpful.

Typically, therapeutic radiopharmaceuticals are administered at standard fixed activities (in gigabecquerel or millicurie), standard fixed activities per unit body mass (MBq kg^{-1}or mCi kg^{-1}) or standard fixed activities per unit body surface area (MBq m^{-2} or mCi m^{-2}) as determined empirically from clinical trials to yield an acceptable maximal frequency or severity of toxicity and an acceptable minimal frequency or extent of therapeutic response. In some cases, the normal tissue toxicity-based approach to prescribing administered activities has been refined by determining the total-body or the critical normal-tissue absorbed dose per unit administered activity (Gy MBq^{-1} or Gy mCi^{-1}) and administering the maximal "safe" activity, that is, the maximal activity that would not deliver a prohibitively toxic normal-tissue absorbed dose. In radioiodine therapy of metastatic thyroid cancer, Benua *et al.* (1962) empirically determined that the maximal "safe" adminis-tered activity generally corresponded to a mean absorbed dose to blood of 2 Gy. As with many therapeutic radiopharmaceuticals, the actual critical, or therapy-limiting, tissue is probably hematopoie-tic red marrow, but the more practically evaluable blood absorbed dose is often used as an index, or surrogate, of the red-marrow absorbed dose. In part because of measurement difficulties (such as relatively coarse spatial resolution, background activity, attenua-tion, and scatter in reliably estimating target-tissue activities and in estimating masses *in vivo* by current radionuclide counting or imaging techniques) the target-tissue absorbed dose per unit administered activity may not be used in prescribing therapeutic administered activities. A notable exception is ^{131}I therapy of Graves disease hyperthyroidism, where some practitioners admin-ister a therapeutic activity projected to deliver an absorbed dose of 70 to 120 Gy to the thyroid. It is possible to do this because doses are based on prior serial thyroid-uptake measurements of a low activity ^{131}I tracer and dosimetric calculations. Almost always, however, it is radiogenic normal-tissue toxicity, and usually mar-row toxicity, that limits and thus dictates the therapeutic adminis-tered activity (Edmonds and Smith, 1986).

Although rarely followed in current practice, an individualized treatment planning paradigm for radiopharmaceutical therapy is generally as follows (Macey *et al.*, 2001; Sgouros, 2005; Siegel *et al.*,

1999; Zanzonico *et al.*, 1995): a low activity "tracer" radiopharmaceutical administration; time activity measurements in target (tumor) and nontarget, normal tissue source regions (*e.g.*, an activity-containing tissue or organ), if possible; absorbed-dose projections in target and nontarget regions, if possible; determination of the maximal "safe" and the minimal "effective" administered activities; and finally the high activity "therapeutic" radiopharmaceutical administration with time activity measurements for determination of the actual therapeutic absorbed doses. It is recommended that the amounts of radiation in radiopharmaceutical therapy be expressed in terms of absorbed dose, and not in terms of administered activity. This recommendation provides a consistent framework for radionuclide therapy based on a standard, radiobiologically significant quantity and incorporates all pertinent patient-specific parameters that can be evaluated practically. However, it requires an accurate assessment of the target tissue masses as well as accurate measurement of time-dependent activities or activity concentrations. To the extent that these quantities are inaccurate, the derived absorbed dose will be inaccurate as well. Despite its utilization in select centers, individualized dose-based treatment planning for radionuclide therapy largely remains an unrealized goal in clinical practice.

The responsibility for prescribing the administered activity for radiopharmaceutical therapy rests with the nuclear-medicine physician. The preparation and administration of therapeutic radiopharmaceuticals *shall* be authorized in writing by the nuclear-medicine physician in the form of a signed prescription. All prescriptions for therapeutic radiopharmaceuticals *shall* contain information unambiguously identifying the patient, the radiopharmaceutical, the activity to be administered, and the route of administration. The prescription may also contain clinical information on the patient's diagnosis and the name of the referring physician, if applicable. The information on the prescription *should* be protected under applicable patient privacy regulations.

3.3.3 *Assay of Administered Activity*

The most common clinical device used to measure the activity in a dosage to be administered to a patient is the so-called "dose calibrator," a sealed, gas-filled, well-type ionization chamber with user-selectable settings specific for various radionuclides. The medical facility shall ensure that this instrument can achieve an accuracy of ±10 % for all therapeutic radionuclides and for all clinically relevant physical forms and geometries of the radionuclides used in the facility (NRC, 2005). For example, a given activity of a therapeutic radionuclide in a solution-filled syringe will generally yield very different readings from the same activity of the same radionuclide in a metallically clad seed for interstitial implantation placed in a vial or test tube. Accordingly, manufacturer-provided or user-derived "correction factors" (*i.e.*, source, volume, and radionuclide-specific calibration factors) may be required. The appropriate correction factor shall be used when assaying the radionuclide dose. Moreover, checks of precision (*i.e.*, reproducibility of serial activity measurements and accuracy checks), or constancy (*i.e.*, checks against an independently calibrated standard source) over the range of photon energies used clinically shall be made prior to first use and on each day of use or clinical operation. The results should be recorded, signed/initialed, and archived. Linearity (*i.e.*, checks of measured versus actual activity over the range of activities used clinically) shall be verified quarterly and the results recorded, signed/initialed, and archived. Tests for accuracy *shall* be performed at least annually using a NIST traceable sealed source. All these checks should be reviewed by a qualified medical physicist or medical health physicist.

The conventional dose calibrator is designed for assay of x- and gamma-ray-emitting radionuclides and is not well suited for assay of radiopharmaceuticals labeled with alpha- or beta-emitting radionuclides. Although energetic beta particles in a relatively high atomic number container may produce sufficient x rays (bremsstrahlung) for detection and assay, the detected signal is highly dependent on the source geometry and the thickness and composition of the container or calibrator. Accordingly, special procedures may need to be developed for the assay of radiopharmaceuticals labeled with alpha or beta emitters. Guidance from the manufacturer or a qualified medical physicist or radiopharmacist *should* be obtained when establishing the specific protocols for assay of such radionuclides. Alternatively, although not routinely available in nuclear-medicine laboratories, beta-emitting radionuclides may be assayed by liquid scintillation counting or other beta counting systems.

There may be difficulties in measuring the activity of alpha-emitting radionuclides if reliance has to be placed completely on alpha counting. However, all of the alpha-emitting radionuclides used therapeutically emit photons of various energies. The calibration, therefore, usually relies on counting of the emitted photons. The services of a qualified medical physicist or medical health physicist *should* be used to set up such calibration systems.

Importantly, regardless of the source and the timing of prior radioassays the activity in each dosage of a radiopharmaceutical *shall* be assayed as close as possible to the time of clinical administration and the results recorded, signed and archived. The residual activity, including that in any intravenous tubing used to administer the dosage, *shall* be assayed promptly after administration so that the actual administered activity can be calculated.

3.3.4 Acceptance Criteria for Therapeutic Radiopharmaceuticals

The identity and quantity of all radioactive and nonradioactive components of any radiopharmaceutical preparation *shall* be known prior to administration to a patient. The manufacturer or supplier *should* provide such a description, typically in the form of a package insert, of the radiopharmaceutical preparation as well as information on shelf-life under specified storage conditions. The ultimate responsibility for the proper administration of radionuclide therapy rests with the nuclear-medicine physician, not with the referring physician or other medical personnel. The attending nuclear-medicine physician *shall* ensure that the composition of the radiopharmaceutical preparation at the time of administration has been established accurately. Other considerations including cost, especially in the case of agents in limited supply, *should not* compel the attending nuclear-medicine physician to administer a suboptimal or inadequately characterized radiopharmaceutical preparation. Information from human and nonhuman toxicology and efficacy studies generally provided by the manufacturer or supplier or information from prior clinical experience *should* be used in such a way that the nuclear-medicine physician can ensure that the radiopharmaceutical is acceptably safe and efficacious for the patient and the condition for which it is being administered. Co-administered solutions and pharmaceutical preparations *shall* be compatible with the radiopharmaceutical and *shall* not significantly reduce its bioavailability by the route administered or alter its expected biodistribution *in vivo*.

Therapeutic radiopharmaceutical preparations shall meet the pharmaceutical criteria set by USP (2004a; 2004b) and FDA. The activity actually administered (*i.e.*, the difference between the gross activity assayed immediately prior to administration and the residual activity assayed immediately after administration) shall be ±10 % of the activity prescribed by the nuclear-medicine physician. For in-house radiopharmaceutical preparations, sufficient QC procedures shall be in place to allow for independent verification by the facility of the pharmaceutical quality and radio-nuclide purity. In large programs, consultation with a pharmacist in the development of these techniques may be required. In addition, parenterally administered radiopharmaceutical preparations shall be isotonic, at physiologic pH, sterile, and pyrogen-free. As noted above, regardless of the source and timing of prior radioassays, the activity in each dosage of a therapeutic radiopharmaceutical preparation shall be assayed as close as possible to the time of the actual administration.

3.3.5 *Administration of Therapeutic Radiopharmaceuticals*

Therapeutic amounts of radiopharmaceuticals *shall* be stored, transported and administered with the use of sufficient shielding so as to maintain personnel exposures ALARA. For orally-administered therapeutic radiopharmaceuticals, the activity-containing vessel *should* be placed in a shielded, spill-proof container with a port, or opening, for the patient to ingest the material, typically drinking a liquid through a straw or taking a capsule. For intravenous use of therapeutic radiopharmaceuticals administered by bolus injection, the activity-containing syringe *should* be placed within a syringe shield with a transparent window that allows visual monitoring of the injectate. For a beta-emitting radionuclide, a plastic syringe shield should be sufficient to reduce hand exposure and minimize the production of bremsstrahlung. For intravenous therapeutic radiopharmaceuticals administered by "slow," or drip, infusion, the activity-containing container, typically an intravenous bag, *should* be placed within a suitable shield. For high-energy photons, such shields will typically be made of a significant thickness of lead such that weight considerations with the stands and measurement devices would need to be evaluated. Intravenous administrations involving the use of infusion pumps would also require shielding the pump, if possible, during the infusion. The advice of the RSO or designee in such decisions is essential.

The procedure for administering a therapeutic radiopharmaceutical *shall* be compatible with its physicochemical properties to ensure as complete a delivery as possible of the prescribed therapeutic activity. For example, certain types of tubing material may adsorb certain radiopharmaceuticals and thereby result in a smaller-than-intended administered activity. Inline filters *shall* be appropriate for and compatible with the radiopharmaceutical. For example, administration of radiolabeled antibodies requires a low-protein-binding filter. It should be noted, however, that filters purposefully retain particulates, including antibody aggregates, and that such retention *shall* be factored into the amount actually delivered into the patient. Syringes, burettes, cups, tubing and other materials used in the administration *should* be flushed or rinsed with isotonic saline (or other physiologic buffer) for parenteral administration. The use of water rinses may be sufficient for oral administration to achieve complete or near-complete administration of the prescribed activity to the patient. All materials resulting from such administrations *shall* be considered as medical and radioactive waste and stored in an appropriate manner (see Section 2 for a brief discussion of radioactive waste disposal methods).

Immediately prior to administration of a therapeutic radiopharmaceutical, the following information, as applicable, *should* be verified by two individuals:

- dose on the radiopharmaceutical label matches the prescription;
- identification of the patient by two independent means;
- identity of radionuclide;
- identity of radiopharmaceutical;
- total activity;
- date and time of calibration; and
- precautions to be followed.

The administered activity *should* be verified in a dose calibrator or other suitable device to ensure that the total activity does not deviate from the prescribed administered activity by >10 %. After administration of the therapeutic radiopharmaceutical, the residual activity in the syringe, cups, tubing, inline filter, or other materials used in the administration *should* be assayed so that corrections to administered activity can be calculated.

To avoid administration of a therapeutic radiopharmaceutical to the wrong patient, the identity of the patient *should* be verified verbally with the patient and checked by a second independent method. Patient identification errors can result from simple problems, such as difficulty in comprehension of the spoken language, or from more complex problems, such as problems of physical impairment (visual, auditory or mental states) due to medication(s). The second verification method *shall* be sufficiently sophisticated to eliminate problems of patients with the same or similar names (*e.g.*, the use of social security number, photo identifications, etc.). As necessary, the services of a translator *should* be obtained for patients whose comprehension of spoken English inhibits their consent or understanding. For inpatients, the identity of the patient *should* also be verified by crosschecking the requisition and the patient's wristband and chart. A therapeutic radiopharmaceutical *shall* never be administered to a patient whose identity cannot be definitively verified.

3.3.6 *Addressable Events*

An addressable event may be considered to be any clinical or technical event that occurs in the course of planning, executing or managing a radiopharmaceutical therapy procedure which has a significant effect on the safety or efficacy of the procedure and which could have been avoided by appropriate procedural changes. The following are examples of such events:

- administration to a patient of a radiopharmaceutical or radionuclide other than that prescribed;
- administration of a radiopharmaceutical with a radionuclidic or a radiochemical purity less than the applicable specification required by USP or FDA at the time of administration;
- administration of a therapeutic dose of a radiopharmaceutical which deviates from the prescribed dose by >10 %;
- administration of a radiopharmaceutical to a patient other than the intended patient; and
- failure to account for effects on radiopharmaceutical distribution of prior, concurrent or subsequently prescribed medication(s), solutions, or medical procedures which may compromise therapeutic efficacy.

Addressable events in radiopharmaceutical therapy *shall* be reported to the RSO and treating physician as soon as they are discovered. The RSO in consultation with the treating physician and the facility administration can then determine if these events meet regulatory standards for reportability. These events *should* also be reported to the patient and the referring physician as soon as possible, preferably within one working day of the discovery. Dose estimates *should* be available to evaluate the absorbed doses to specific organs. The attending nuclear-medicine physician *shall* decide if there would be any expected medical consequences of an event. The dose estimates, timing of further administrations, and clinical effect(s) of the original administration will affect such a decision. Appropriate interventions, such as hydration or attempts to block uptake (*e.g.*, the administration of stable iodides in radioiodinated monoclonal antibody therapy) *shall* be considered in light of the patient's overall medical condition, the medical consequences of the event and the effects of any intervention. Short- and long-term medical management of such events *shall* be planned carefully on an individual basis (NRC, 2004).

Even if an event results in no demonstrable harm to the patient, it may represent a procedural lapse, a breakdown in existing systems, or lead to the identification of systematic problems which need to be addressed. Addressable events may result from human error. However, such a finding should not preclude consideration of factors that contribute to these errors, including the workload of the individual, staffing issues, and the working environment. Certain addressable events may meet the criteria for reporting to regulatory agencies. A careful analysis *shall* be performed to determine the cause or causes of the event. This analysis *should* include interviews of involved personnel, reviews of pertinent policies and procedures, reviews of training, and consideration of any other relevant factors. A plan for actions to prevent a recurrence *should* be developed; these actions *should* address the causes identified by the causal analysis (NRC, 2005). If appropriate, remediation, including further education of personnel or development of further safeguards, *should* be implemented.

3.3.7 *Considerations in Patient Confinement*

In considering the release or confinement of patients during and after treatment, the nuclear-medicine physician *shall* determine that the patient is willing and is physically and mentally able to comply with appropriate radiation safety precautions in the medical facility should medical confinement be necessary or at home after release. Other factors affecting this decision are discussed in Section 3.4. Importantly, if the nuclear-medicine physician determines that the patient is unwilling or unable to comply and would, therefore, pose a radiation hazard to the staff of the medical facility and others, radiopharmaceutical therapy may be withheld and alternative treatments considered. If the nuclear-medicine physician determines that a patient, despite difficulties, may nonetheless be safely treated with appropriate and reasonable medical supervision while hospitalized, patient treatment may proceed. The nuclear-medicine physician can determine that such patients can and *should* remain hospitalized beyond the period of time dictated by any other criteria. As an example, for an incontinent patient, the nuclear-medicine physician may determine that hospitalization of the patient be extended to ensure safe collection and disposal of radioactively contaminated urine. Both the radiological and clinical considerations *shall* be given due weight by the nuclear-medicine physician. These considerations are discussed further in Section 3.4 and Appendices A and B.

3.3.8 *Special Considerations for Female Patients*

Deterministic effects can be produced in the human embryo or fetus following irradiation. All of these effects are temporally related to the stage of pregnancy (see Table 4.1 in NCRP, 1994). Because radionuclide therapy typically involves the administration of high activities, typically at gigabecquerel levels, such therapy is generally contraindicated in pregnant women, unless there is no viable alternative. Signs alerting female patients and containing wording similar to, "If you are pregnant or if it is possible you may be pregnant, please notify the staff before the beginning of any procedure," *should* be prominently posted throughout the nuclear-medicine areas, particularly in waiting and dressing areas. A pregnancy test *shall* be performed before radionuclide therapy in any female patient of childbearing age. Assertions by the patient or her family regarding the impossibility of a pregnancy because of medical condition, sexual inactivity, use of birth control measures, or recent menstrual history, should not preclude performing a pregnancy test prior to radionuclide therapy (Zanzonico and Becker, 1991). Physicians and other readers may wish to consult NCRP Commentary No. 9 (NCRP, 1994).

The use of ^{131}I therapy for thyroid diseases in pregnant or potentially pregnant women is particularly problematic because radiogenic destruction of the iodine-avid fetal thyroid may result from such treatment and could cause hypothyroidism *in utero* and cretinism. The fetal thyroid begins concentrating iodine at the 12th to 15th week of gestation and fetal absorbed doses can be >10 Gy per 37 MBq administered to the mother, depending on gestational age and maternal thyroid uptake. Therapeutic administered activities of 0.37 to 3.7 GBq of iodine would, therefore, result in fetal thyroid absorbed doses from 100 to 1,000 Gy, respectively. Case reports that include administered activity, gestational age, and follow-up of pregnant women treated with radioiodine for hyperthyroidism or thyroid cancer indicate that the outcome of pregnancy with regard to fetal thyroid function at birth did not appear to be compromised in the cases when radioiodine was given before the 10th week of pregnancy. However, there was essentially a 100 % occurrence of congenital hypothyroidism or cretinism when radioiodine was administered thereafter, even in amounts <5 GBq (Zanzonico and

Becker, 1991). Pregnancy is a contraindication to radioiodine therapy and, as stated above, a pregnancy test *shall* be performed before administration of such therapy in any female patient of childbearing age.

Virtually any systemically administered material, including a therapeutic radiopharmaceutical, will appear to some extent in the milk of a lactating female. Radiopharmaceuticals will, therefore, be transferred to and irradiate a breastfed infant. The generally high administered activities of therapeutic radiopharmaceuticals may result in relatively high activity concentrations in milk and ingestion, cumulatively, of relatively high activities by the infant. Moreover, because of their small size and the inverse relationship between absorbed dose and mass, ingestion of even a relatively small amount of activity by an infant will result in proportionately large total body and organ absorbed doses. Further, because of proximity of the infant to the mother when nursing, there is a potentially significant external absorbed dose to the infant. It is the responsibility of the administering physician, typically the nuclear-medicine physician, to ascertain if a patient is nursing a child by breast prior to administration of a therapeutic radiopharmaceutical. Accordingly, nursing is generally a contraindication to radiopharmaceutical therapy and *shall* be discontinued prior to radiopharmaceutical therapy. The duration of the cessation of nursing will depend on the radionuclide and its effective half-life *in vivo*, the administered activity, and the extent to which the radionuclide is concentrated in breast milk. For those who choose, breast milk may be collected with a breast pump and refrigerated for several days before administration of a therapeutic radiopharmaceutical. Based on radioassay of serial milk samples expressed with a breast pump, nursing may be resumed when the breast milk is no longer detectably radioactive except in the case of ^{131}I as discussed below. Signs alerting women with language such as, "If you are breastfeeding, please notify the staff before the beginning of any procedure," *should* be prominently posted in the nuclear-medicine areas, particularly in waiting and dressing areas. Where facilities serve non-English speaking populations, signs in the appropriate languages *should* also be posted.

Iodine-131 therapy of thyroid disease in nursing mothers presents particular problems because of the relatively long physical half-life (8 d) and the significant localization of radioiodine in their milk and the resulting high thyroid absorbed dose in infants. Accordingly, nursing by women who have received therapeutic amounts of ^{131}I *shall* be discontinued permanently for a baby who is currently nursing, as it is impractical to expect a mother to resume nursing after discontinuing nursing for up to several months.

The majority of radiopharmaceutical therapy, by far, is in the form of [131]I. The sodium-iodide symporter protein, which actively transports iodide across the cell membrane, is found not only in the thyroid gland but also in other tissues, particularly lactating mammary glands (Spitzweg and Morris, 2002). The role of sodium-iodide symporter in the mammary gland is to actively transport iodide into the milk, thereby supplying iodide to the infant. The length of time required for down-regulation of sodium-iodide symporter protein production in mammary tissue after cessation of breastfeeding varies but has been reported in some cases to be in excess of five weeks (Hsiao *et al.*, 2004). Administration of ^{131}I too soon after cessation of breastfeeding both increases the radiation dose to the radiosensitive breast tissue of the woman as well as complicates the interpretation of the images acquired (Bakheet *et al.*, 1998). Because of the localization of radioiodine in breast tissue as well as breast milk, assessment of the breastfeeding status of the woman *shall* be made prior to scheduling treatment. Accordingly, nursing by women who will receive or have received therapeutic amounts of [131]I *shall* be discontinued permanently for a baby who is currently nursing.

For female patients who may be menstruating during or immediately after a therapeutic administration, there may be detectable contamination on pads or tampons. Local regulations may differ regarding disposal of these items. It is recommended that these items be collected for the first 1 to 3 d post-administration and be held for decay to background levels prior to proper disposal.

3.3.9 *Heritable Effects and Genetic Counseling*

Even after comprehensive studies of well over 10,000 children born to the atomic-bomb survivors in Hiroshima and Nagasaki with mean gonadal doses of >0.3 Gy, there remains no direct evidence for heritable radiation effects in humans. The estimation of human genetic risks is, therefore, based largely on data derived from laboratory studies in animals, introducing the considerable uncertainty of extrapolation from nonhuman systems to humans. The total risk per gray per million progeny of the first generation as a percent of baseline is from 0.41 to 0.64 (NAS/NRC, 2006).

Although the numbers of patients are small, several studies have generally demonstrated little or no radiogenic germ-cell mutagenesis among thyroid cancer patients treated with large amounts of [131]I (Edmonds and Smith, 1986; Sarkar *et al.*, 1976).

The absorbed dose to the gonads for ^{131}I therapy is relatively low (*i.e.*, <1 Gy) for administered activities of several gigabecquerel (Zanzonico, 1997). In view of these doses, the high threshold for the induction of permanent sterility in human beings (*i.e.*, 3.5 Gy for the testis and 2.5 Gy for the ovary) and the low risk factors for radiogenic germ-cell damage, it is not surprising that there is a general absence of impaired fertility and of birth defects among subsequently conceived children of ^{131}I therapy patients (NAS/ NRC, 2006). Nonetheless, demonstrable but transient gonadal damage, such as impaired fertility based on sperm counts over the first year post-treatment, may occur among ^{131}I therapy patients (Edmonds and Smith, 1986; Handelsman and Turtle, 1983). Follow-up studies of such patients indicate that among male patients there is a time dependent recovery of sperm count. This may take as long as 2 y in some cases. Longer-term studies (*i.e.*, 10 y or longer post-treatment among both male and female patients) indicate that fertility and the frequencies of miscarriages and congenital abnormalities among their offspring are comparable to control values. Collectively these findings are generally consistent with the results of the seminal studies of Russell and associates in male and female mice (Russell, 1977; Russell and Kelly, 1982). The general consensus is that males *should* forego fathering children for at least six months after high-dose radioiodine therapy and females *should* avoid becoming pregnant for 12 months after such therapy. The rationale for the waiting period for males, in addition to allowing for the physical decay of ^{131}I, is that ^{131}I therapy has been found to be associated with transient impairment of testicular germinal cell function and any damaged spermatozoon are replaced after four months (Hyer *et al.*, 2002; Pacini *et al.*, 1994). For females, the waiting period allows the body to regain normal hormonal balance that contributes to a more successful pregnancy and allows confirmation of complete disease remission with follow-up scans (often performed with ^{131}I) at 12 months post-therapy (Casara *et al.*, 1993; Schlumberger *et al.*, 1996). Follow-up scans would, of course, be problematic if the patient were pregnant. These waiting periods would also avoid the frustration caused by possible transient impairment of fertility. Accordingly, following high activity radiopharmaceutical therapy, male patients and female patients *should* be advised to forego attempting to have children for at least 6 and 12 months post-therapy, respectively. Some patients may wish to consider the possibility of sperm banking and other techniques based on their individual situations, and genetic counseling services *should* be available to patients wishing to pursue these options.

3.4 Radiation Safety Procedures

These procedures *should* be considered supplemental to the radiation safety program requirements discussed in Section 2. Operational radiation safety is also discussed in NCRP Report No. 105, Report No. 127, and Report No. 134 (NCRP 1989; 1998; 2000) and Siegel (2004) as well as documents issued by other professional scientific organizations.

Decisions as to whether or not physicians, nurses and other personnel caring for or working in the vicinity of radioactive patients are to be classified as radiation workers are to be made by the RSO in consultation with facility management and the RSC. To minimize exposure of personnel, it is generally recommended that patients receiving therapeutic amounts of activity not be concentrated in one area or treated at one time but dispersed spatially and temporally (if clinically acceptable). However, there are circumstances where such dispersal may not be possible and it may be necessary to concentrate patients in designated areas under care of specially trained, experienced personnel. Such decisions are a matter of facility policy and *should* involve consultation with the RSO to ascertain that the ALARA principle is maintained. Pregnant women *shall not* be responsible for the routine care of patients receiving therapeutic amounts of radiopharmaceuticals.

Generally, there is no need to isolate or otherwise limit access to patients who have received radiopharmaceutical therapy with a beta emitter. Standard precautions *should* be used with these patients. However, there may be special circumstances, as with marrow ablative therapy, where the potential for contamination is significant. With such patients the RSO *should* ensure that the staff is given special instruction in the procedures to be followed. Special care *should* be taken to avoid the possibility of beta emitters coming in contact with the skin of the caregiver, especially if such emitters have the potential to bind with chemicals in the body. In the event that residual contamination is determined to be present, immediate decontamination *should* proceed until the residual contamination is reduced to a level acceptable to the RSO.

Unless otherwise specified by the RSO, nurses, physicians and other health care personnel are to perform all routine duties, including those requiring direct patient contact, in a normal manner but personnel *should* avoid lingering near the patient unnecessarily. Patients *should* be apprised in advance of the necessity for medical personnel to minimize close or direct contact so that this precaution will not be interpreted as a lack of concern. To the extent possible, verbal communication with the patients *should* be conducted from a distance (*e.g.*, the doorway to a room). Housekeeping, food service, and other ancillary personnel *should* likewise perform all essential routine tasks expeditiously and *should* avoid entering the patient's room for nonessential tasks. In an inpatient setting, ancillary personnel *should not* enter the patient's room without conferring with the nursing staff. Personnel caring for such a patient or otherwise entering the room *should* observe standard precautions and thoroughly wash their hands after leaving the patient's room. In selected cases, persons entering the room of a patient may be asked to don protective clothing before entering and to leave such clothing in the area after exiting the room. These precautions are to be decided on an individual basis by the facility RSO.

Patients who require hospitalization may have visitors during the period that radiation precautions are in effect. In addition, a member of a patient's family may be permitted to receive up to 50 mSv y^{-1} on the recommendation of the treating physician. When family members are likely to receive dose >5 mSv annually, they *should* be provided training and individual monitoring as if they were to be occupationally exposed (NCRP, 1995b). When in the opinion of the treating physician, there are significant extenuating reasons to allow members of the family to exceed the dose limitations of Table 2.1, consultation *shall* be sought with the RSO to see if the use of portable shielding or limitations on visiting times can mitigate any potential dose. Special attention *shall* be given to limitations on the doses to pregnant women and children. Every reasonable effort *shall* be made to reduce the doses received by pregnant women and children. The design of specific rooms for housing patients receiving radiopharmaceutical therapy is discussed in Section 5.

A patient receiving a therapeutic administration of a radiopharmaceutical and requiring medical confinement according to the foregoing criteria *shall* be placed in a private hospital room with a private toilet and sink. The nuclear-medicine physician *should* arrange with the admitting office for this type of room to be available immediately prior to administration and for the duration of the admission. The nuclear-medicine physician *should* convey the date of the treatment, the radionuclide, the radiopharmaceutical, and the prescribed administered activity to the RSO as far in advance as possible. The nuclear-medicine physician and the RSO *should* decide in advance whether or not the patient is suitable for release on the same day that the radiopharmaceutical therapy is administered (Sparks *et al.*, 1998). Any limitations for same-day release will depend on facility and medical decisions but can include consideration of:

- type of dwelling;
- presence in the household of pregnant or breastfeeding women;
- sex and age of each household member;
- sleeping partner information;
- information on children in the household;
- workplace information and schedule;
- presence in the workplace of pregnant women or minors;
- means of transportation from hospital to home;
- physical challenges;
- incontinence or ostomy care; and
- ability to comprehend instructions.

The discussion in the remainder of this Section assumes that the patient requires confinement in a medical facility. For a discussion regarding same-day treatment and release without confinement, see Appendices A and B.

On the day of the planned treatment, the patient's hospital room *should* be prepared to minimize potential radioactive contamination. The use of disposable plastic-backed absorbent pads taped in place in the areas most likely to be contaminated, such as the floor around the toilet and sink, is one option used in many facilities. The therapeutic radiopharmaceutical, activity, the date and time of administration, and verification of the assay *shall* be entered in some form in the patient's medical record. Prior to administration of the therapeutic radiopharmaceutical to the patient, all radiation safety precautions *shall* be explained to the patient. If the administration requires admission to the facility, the patient *should* clearly understand the necessity to stay in the assigned room and the limitations on visiting time to avoid any anxiety. This explanation *should* take place prior to admission to the facility so that any questions from the patient can be addressed in a timely manner and the patient's anxiety, if any, relieved. A signed and dated copy of the radiation safety precautions *should* be placed in the patient's medical record. Any contaminated items from the procedure *should* be labeled with the radionuclide, a radiation precaution sticker, and held for complete decay in storage in an appropriately shielded and secure area. In practical terms, this will mean holding material until there is no measurable activity. Federal or local regulations *should* also be consulted for specific requirements.

Anterior exposure rates at the surface of and 1 m from the patient *should* be measured at the level of the patient's umbilicus, using a calibrated radiation monitor, such as a portable ionization chamber. These initial measurements *should* be performed within 1 h of administration of the radiopharmaceutical therapy and prior to any post-therapy excretion by the patient. The radionuclide, the radiopharmaceutical, and the activity administered *shall* also be recorded in the patient's medical record. A "radiation precautions" sign *should* be posted on the door to the patient's room and a "radioactive precautions" wristband placed on the patient's wrist.

There *should* be available in the patient's room a plastic or plastic-lined container for short-term disposal/storage of all disposable items used by the patient. Food and beverages for the patient *should* be provided using disposable trays, cups, utensils, etc. The patient may use the toilet and dispose of urine and feces as usual, flushing the toilet several times after each use. The patient's linens and gowns may also be contaminated and *should* be held for checks by the radiation safety staff before being placed in the facility laundry. In practical terms this will mean holding linen until there is no measurable activity. Federal or local regulations *should* be consulted for specific requirements.

Each day following administration of the therapeutic radiopharmaceutical, the patient *should* be resurveyed. The point at which these surveys are made *should* be the area of maximal uptake of the radiopharmaceutical. Scans of the patient's body with a survey meter may be necessary to find the area of maximal uptake. For example, in the case of thyroid treatments in patients with intact thyroids, this area may correspond to the patient's neck or chest. The exposure rate measured can then be used to determine release instructions for the patient, if any. Removal of contaminated items from the patient's room *should* be done on a daily basis.

Upon discharge of the patient, the RSO *should* arrange for removal of all remaining waste and contaminated items from the patient's hospital room. All items *should* be placed in plastic bags, using separate bags for disposable and for nondisposable items (*e.g.,* linens and bedding). All radioactively contaminated items *should* be labeled with radiation precaution stickers and with the radionuclide, date and time, and held for decay-in-storage in an appropriate shielded and secure area until there is no measurable activity. All waste and other items being held for decay in storage *should* be reassayed periodically using a calibrated radiation monitor. Waste *should* then be discarded appropriately and bedding and linens may be treated as usual.

The patient's room *shall* be surveyed and checked for removable contamination. Initially, this check *should* be performed using a handheld survey meter, such as a GM counter or scintillation survey meter. These checks *should* be followed as necessary with wipe testing. When the applicable criteria for removable radioactive contamination specified by the RSO are satisfied, the medical facility *should* be informed that the room is available for general patient use.

A list of names and 24 h telephone numbers of individuals to contact in the event of a radiation emergency *shall* be available. This list is separate in function from listings of persons responding to radiation emergencies in emergency rooms or trauma centers. Personnel to be contacted may include the RSO and responsible nuclear-medicine physician or the nuclear-medicine resident or fellow on-call. These lists *shall* be available to medical personnel caring for the patient. Specific instructions for emergency situations are given in Section 6.

In the event of a large volume spill of blood, urine or vomitus, nursing personnel *should* cover the spill with a plastic-backed absorbent pad and immediately call the designated radiation safety staff. For inpatients that received regional radiopharmaceutical therapy, spills from these patients will usually contain minimal activity. Medical personnel *should not* attempt to clean up a major spill without radiation safety instruction.

3.5 Patient-Release Criteria

The release criteria for patients receiving therapeutic amounts of radiopharmaceuticals are based on the prevailing recommendations promulgated in NCRP Report No. 116 (NCRP, 1993b) and NCRP Commentary 11 (NCRP, 1995b). This Section is supplementary to the discussion in Section 3.3.5 and incorporates recommendations previously presented in NCRP Report No. 37 (NCRP, 1970). A discussion of the operational equations governing patient release and examples of their applications can be found in Appendices A and B (Zanzonico, 1997; 2000). Regulatory agencies have published criteria for patient release and these criteria *shall* be reviewed by the RSO and the nuclear-medicine physician(s) in facilities administering therapeutic amounts of radiopharmaceuticals to determine which criteria apply to the facility-specific program (NRC, 1987; 1997; 2002; 2005).

3.5.1 *Doses to Individuals and Family Members*

NCRP Report No. 37 and Commentary No. 11 (NCRP, 1970; 1993b) recommended an annual dose limit of 5 mSv annually for family members caring for or living with persons treated with therapeutic amounts of radiopharmaceuticals. This recommendation was based on the consideration that caring for such individuals most likely represented an once-in-a-lifetime circumstance for the family member(s). The recommendations required that instruction be provided to the family member(s) regarding any limitations on living circumstances, such as sleeping arrangements or care for small children. These considerations are discussed in Appendices A and B. There have been a number of reports on the contamination potential for both the premises occupied by the patients and individuals caring for these patients (Barrington et al., 1996; 1999; Buchanan and Brindle, 1970; 1971; Grigsby et al., 2000; Harbert and Wells, 1974; Jacobson et al., 1978; Macle et al., 1999; Mathieu et al., 1999; Miller, 1992; Rutar et al., 2001a; 2001b; Ryan et al., 2000; Siegel, 1998; Siegel and Rutar, 2002; Zanzonico et al., 1999). Virtually all of these authors have reached the conclusion that the release of patients treated with therapeutic amounts of radiopharmaceuticals is not likely to expose any member of the public, inclusive of both external and internal dose contributions, >5 mSv provided that adequate instructions are provided at discharge to the patient and the family members.

3.5.2 *Travel by Radiopharmaceutical Therapy Patients*

An important practical issue with radiopharmaceutical therapy patients is limitation of travel, because this will typically involve exposure from the patient to one or more individuals at relatively close distances in a confined space, such as an automobile or airplane. Various authors have reported measurable dose rates at 0.1 to 1 m from ^{131}I treated hyperthyroid and thyroid cancer patients immediately post-administration (Barrington et al., 1996; Culver and Dworkin, 1991; Gunasekera et al., 1996; Pochin and Kermode, 1975). While it is difficult to succinctly summarize these data, traveling with a patient for 1 h following administration of ^{131}I is unlikely to result in an effective dose >1 mSv at a distance 0.3 m or further from a patient who received an activity of the order of 370 MBq or at a distance 1 m or further from a patient who received an activity of the order of 3.7 GBq. However, in the case of administered activities at the latter level and at distances from the patient of 0.3 m or less, an effective dose >5 mSv may be accrued >1 h. Thus, travel for 1 h immediately post-treatment in a private automobile large enough for a patient to maintain a distance of 1 m or greater from the other occupant(s) is generally permissible. However, a case-by-case analysis will be necessary to determine the actual travel restrictions for each patient, especially for longer trips and for travel by public bus or train, commercial airliner, or other conveyance in which travelers may be crowded together.

Patients containing small amounts of radiopharmaceuticals can cause an alarm from sensitive radiation detectors used at airports, train stations, and other locations. Patients *should* be aware of this possibility and *should* have a letter or card, containing the appropriate information, issued by the treating institution for display to authorities. Such a card or letter *should* include a method of verifying this information with the treating facility.

3.6 Emerging Applications

Algorithms for patient-specific dosimetry suitable for radiopharmaceutical therapy treatment planning are not yet widely available (Zanzonico, 2000). As a result, "dose prescription" algorithms in radiopharmaceutical therapy remain relatively simple:

- administration of the same activity to all patients;
- administration of activity per unit body mass or surface area (MBq kg^{-1} or MBq m^{-2}) to all patients; or
- administration of the patient-specific activity corresponding to some empirically determined maximal tolerated dose (*e.g.*, 2 Gy to the blood, as a bone marrow surrogate, in ^{131}I-sodium-iodide treatment of metastatic thyroid cancer (Zanzonico, 2000; Zanzonico *et al.*, 1995).

The tumor dose is generally not determined and thus is not used for treatment planning. However, with the application of quantitative positron-emission tomography (PET) imaging, as illustrated by the use of ^{124}I-iodide in thyroid cancer (Pentlow *et al.*, 1991; 1996; Sgouros *et al.*, 2004), the procedures may be changing. PET and, in particular, combined PET/computed tomography (CT) is among the most rapidly expanding areas in nuclear medicine (Schoder *et al.*, 2003). At present, PET systems employing detector elements numbering in the thousands, septa-less three-dimensional data acquisition and iterative image reconstruction are yielding quantitative whole-body images with a spatial resolution of ~5 mm or better in <30 min (Zanzonico, 2004). Manufacturers are now also marketing multi-modality scanners, combining high-performance state-of-the-art PET and CT scanners in a single device. These devices provide near-perfect registration of images of *in vivo* function (PET) and anatomy (CT) and are already having a major impact on clinical practice, particularly in oncology (Schoder *et al.*, 2003).

Another burgeoning area in nuclear medicine is the application of intraoperative probes, particularly in the detection and localization of so-called "sentinel" lymph nodes in breast cancer and in melanoma (Cody, 2002; Zanzonico and Heller, 2000).

Radiopharmaceutical therapies, most notably radioimmunotherapy, peptide therapy, and palliation of malignant bone pain, continue to be areas of intensive investigation. Recently, FDA approved two radiolabeled anti-CD20 antibodies, Bexxar® (labeled with ^{131}I; Corixa, Seattle, Washington) and Zevalin® (labeled with ^{90}Y), for treatment of non-Hodgkin's B-cell lymphomas (Gates et al., 1998; Meredith, 2006; Witzig, 2006). Both agents have proven effective for relapsed and refractory low-grade and transformed lymphomas and have renewed interest in radioimmunotherapy of solid tumors (Jhanwar and Divgi, 2005; Pandit-Taskar et al., 2003; 2004). The development of immune constructs [from polyclonal antibodies to murine monoclonal antibodies to chimeric antibodies (composed of a human constant region fused with a murine variable region) to humanized antibodies (composed of an antigen-binding region or complementarity-determining region on a human immunoglobulin structure)] not only improves tumor targeting but reduces the antibody's immunogenicity and, therefore, the development of human anti-mouse antibodies. In addition, improvement of penetration into solid tumor parenchyma and clearance from normal tissues is being pursued by the use of smaller immune constructs than intact immunoglobulins. These include Fab' and F(ab)'^{2} fragments and, more recently, single-chain antigen binding proteins (sFv) (linear constructs of light and heavy Fv fragments rapidly cleared from blood and having lower renal retention compared to Fab' fragments), two sFv fragments linked by a component of the heavy-chain regions, and dia-bodies (two covalently linked sFv fragments). To further enhance the efficacy of radioimmunotherapy, multi-step (or pre-) targeting strategies are being actively investigated. These are designed to minimize the radiation dose to normal tissue due to prolonged residence time in the body while not significantly reducing tumor targeting. One widely investigated approach utilizes the ultra-high-affinity interaction between avidin (or streptavidin) and biotin. The nonradioactive targeting antibody or fragment is conjugated with avidin or streptavidin before injection. Approximately 1 d thereafter, a clearing agent is administered to reduce the amount of the nonradioactive antibody-(streptavidin) avidin complex remaining in the circulation and normal tissues prior to administration of the radiolabeled biotin. Finally, the radiolabeled biotin is injected and rapidly either binds the radionuclide to the (streptavidin) avidin in the tumor or is excreted. Originally, antibodies and antibody fragments were radiolabeled exclusively with radioiodines such as ^{123}I or, more commonly, [131]I. More recently, various chelates are being used to bind a variety of radiometals such as ^{90}Y and ^{177}Lu to these agents (Bander *et al.*, 2003).

Peptide-based radiopharmaceuticals were introduced clinically more than a decade ago, with the somatostatin analog, octreotide, used for both receptor scintigraphy (with ^{111}In label) and also receptor-mediated peptide radiotherapy with either ^{111}In or ^{90}Y as the radiolabel of neuroendocrine tumors, remaining the most successful and widely used of these agents (Gotthardt *et al.*, 2004). Such a peptide must generally be modified with a radiometal chelator complex to allow stable labeling with a so-called residualizing label, meaning that the radiometal-chelator-peptide complex is internalized *via* a specific receptor and trapped in target cells. In addition to octreotide, peptides under development for use as radiopharmaceuticals include minigastrin, substance P, and neurotensin.

Potentially debilitating bone pain resulting from skeletal metastases is a common feature of many advanced cancers, such as prostate and breast cancer. While ERT remains the principal approach for pain palliation for solitary skeletal lesions, bone-seeking radiopharmaceuticals are widely used for treatment of multiple painful osseous lesions (Pandit-Taskar *et al.*, 2004). Although ^{32}P was used for many years, its associated myelosuppression has led to the ongoing development of other bone-seeking radiopharmaceuticals, including ^{89}Sr-labeled strontium chloride ([89]SrCl), [153]Sm-labeled ethylenediaminetetramethylene phosphonic acid ([153]Sm-EDTMP), [117m]Sn-labeled stannous chloride ([117m]SnCl), and [166]Ho-labeled 1,4,7,10-tetraazacyclododecane-1,4,7,10-tetramethylenephosphonate ([166]Ho-DOTMP). Currently, [89]SrCl and [153]Sm-EDTMP have been approved by FDA for the treatment of painful osseous metastases.

The use of ^{90}Y labeled microspheres for the treatment of liver cancers has been approved by FDA. Patients with metastatic liver tumors, primarily from colorectal cancers, represent the largest group of patients treated using ^{90}Y-microsphere techniques. However, some centers have elected to use this technique for treatment of primary liver cancers (Herba *et al.*, 1988; Lim *et al.*, 2005; Stubbs *et al.*, 2001; Welsh, 2006). Yttrium-90 microspheres have been used with and without concomitant chemotherapy. Although technically a form of brachytherapy, the necessity for a hepatic arteriogram and arterial embolization, have resulted in most of these procedures being performed in an interventional radiology setting; an area in most facilities where therapeutic treatment with radionuclides has not been previously used. Typical administered activities have varied from 1 to 3 GBq. Physicians administering the doses may be nuclear-medicine physicians rather than radiation oncologists. Refer to Section 4.9 for a discussion of the brachytherapy techniques that may apply. Personnel administering these activities *should* be instructed in the use of plastic shields and plastic syringe shields, some of which may be supplied by the pharmaceutical manufacturer (Murthy *et al.*, 2005a; Salem, 2006). Various techniques, including bremsstrahlung imaging, have been developed to analyze the distribution of the microspheres following placement (Campbell *et al.*, 2000). The success of this technique reported to date will possibly lead to the expansion of this use to other tumors.

4. Brachytherapy

4.1 Techniques and Basic Terminology

Brachytherapy is a technique that places sealed radioactive sources adjacent to or in contact with a target tissue. Because the absorbed dose falls off rapidly with increasing distance from the sources, high doses (3 to 70 Gy) may be safely delivered to a well-localized target or region over a short time period; typically from a few minutes up to one week for temporary implants and a period from several days to several months for permanent implants. The procedure of surgically inserting sealed radioactive sources or placement of catheters or applicators designed to hold them is known as "implantation." The term "implant" usually refers to a completed assembly of sources with or without applicators used for therapeutic intent. Some techniques for regional therapy are discussed in Section 3.

Implantation techniques may be classified by a variety of methods. In terms of the surgical approach to the target volume, implants may be termed as interstitial, intracavitary, transluminal or techniques employing molds. If one designates the means of controlling the dose delivered, implants may be temporary or permanent. Classification in terms of source-loading technology results in terms such as preloaded, manually afterloaded, or remotely afterloaded. Finally, techniques can be defined by the dose rate employed: low, medium or high.

Intracavitary insertion consists of positioning applicators, bearing appropriate sources, into a body cavity in proximity to the target tissue. Intracavitary treatment is almost universally used in definitive radiation therapy of locally advanced cervical cancer. All intracavitary implants are temporary implants that are removed from the patient as soon as the prescribed dose has been delivered. The vaginal cylinder is the most commonly used intracavitary surface-dose applicator in gynecologic brachytherapy.

Interstitial brachytherapy consists of surgically implanting small sealed radioactive sources, also called "seeds," directly into target tissues. Temporary interstitial implants consist of sealed radioactive sources placed into steel needles or plastic catheters that are inserted in the target tissue and that are removed at the end of a precalculated treatment or "dwell" time. A permanent

71

interstitial implant remains in place for the lifetime of the individual or until coincidentally removed during surgery. The initial source strength is chosen so that the prescribed dose is fully delivered only when the implanted radioactive material has decayed to a negligible level. Surface-dose application (sometimes called plesiocurie or mold therapy) consists of an applicator, which may be customized to individual patient contours, containing an array of sealed radioactive sources designed to deliver a uniform dose distribution to skin or a mucosal surface. Transluminal brachytherapy consists of inserting a single line source into a body lumen to treat its surface and adjacent tissues.

Temporary implant technology can be classified in terms of the method used to introduce, or load, the sealed radioactive sources into the implant site. The preloaded or "hot source" technique consists of placing the sealed radioactive sources directly, or placing applicators previously loaded with sources, in the implant site during an operative procedure. Since 1970, most temporary implants are implemented by using manually afterloaded applicator systems. Nonradioactive or unloaded applicators are inserted into the patient during an operative procedure. The sealed radioactive sources are subsequently "afterloaded" into the applicator system when the patient has returned to his or her room. These techniques, introduced into practice during the early 1960s, eliminate exposure to operating room personnel and to the hands and fingers of the radiation oncologist (Henscke et al., 1963; Suit et al., 1963). For intracavitary therapy, tube-like sources of ^{137}Cs (sometimes called "intracavitary tubes") are manually manipulated into plastic sleeves or inserts that are then introduced into vaginal and uterine applicators as indicated. For temporary interstitial implants, flexible plastic tubes or hollow metal needles are inserted into the target tissue during an operative procedure. After the patient has returned to his or her room, ribbons containing sealed radioactive sources are inserted into the hollow applicators. These techniques are discussed in Section 4.2.2 (see Figure 4.1 for source types).

Radiation exposure to hospital staff responsible for source loading and the care of implant patients during treatment can be greatly reduced or eliminated by use of remote afterloading technology (Glasgow, 1995b). A remote afterloading system consists of a pneumatically or motor-driven source transport system for robotically transferring radioactive material between a shielded safe and each treatment site. The applicators or catheters are connected to a shielded safe by means of transfer tubes. Most remote afterloaders are equipped with a timer that automatically retracts the sources when the programmed treatment time, corrected for gaps

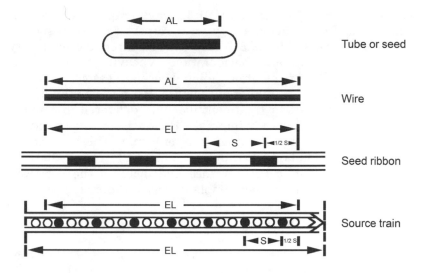

Fig. 4.1. The types of brachytherapy sources shown reflect current usage in the United States. *AL* is the active length, *EL* is the equivalent active length, and *S* is the separation between small sources (ICRU, 1997).

and interruptions, has been administered. Use of these devices is reviewed in more detail later in this Section.

The rate at which absorbed dose is delivered to the treatment site (prescription dose rate) greatly influences the logistics of treatment delivery, the radiation safety procedures necessary, and the patient's response to treatment. According to the conventions of ICRU Report 38 (ICRU, 1985), dose rates of 0.4 to 2 Gy h^{-1} at the prescription point are referred to as low dose-rate (LDR) implants. To deliver clinically useful total doses of 10 to 70 Gy, treatment times of 24 to 144 h are required. This requirement limits the practice of LDR brachytherapy to the inpatient environment. The total source strength loaded in LDR implants results in low exposure rates around the patient. Even with manual afterloading techniques, good quality nursing and medical care can be administered without exceeding acceptable limits for exposure of personnel. The vast bulk of accumulated clinical brachytherapy experience consists of retrospective studies of patients treated using LDR techniques. Using the ICRU conventions, an HDR implant is one utilizing prescription dose rates >0.2 Gy min^{-1} (>12 Gy h^{-1}) (ICRU, 1985). Modern HDR remote afterloaders contain sources capable of delivering dose rates as high as 0.12 Gy s^{-1} at 1 cm distance in tissue. Treatment times are typically of the order of minutes. As

discussed later in this Section, HDR brachytherapy differs significantly from LDR brachytherapy with respect to dose response,
level of technical and logistical complexity required, patient safety
issues, and socio-economic considerations. A heavily shielded treatment room and a remote afterloading device are essential components of an HDR brachytherapy facility. HDR brachytherapy is
generally an outpatient treatment modality delivered in discrete
fractions at daily or weekly intervals. From two to eight fractions
of HDR treatment are required to approximate the tumoricidal
effect of LDR implant therapy. An ultra-LDR range (0.01 to
0.3 Gy h^{-1}) is of clinical importance and includes the dose-rate
domain utilized by permanent implants using low-energy seeds.

4.2 Sources, Delivery Technology, and Dosimetry

Classically, "sealed" brachytherapy sources consist of a core that
is coated or impregnated with a radioactive material. This core is
then sealed in a metal sheath or capsule, typically titanium
for low-energy photon sources and stainless steel or platinum for
higher-energy photon sources. Encapsulation prevents leakage of
radioactive material and absorbs nonpenetrating radiation (*i.e.*,
alpha and beta radiations and very-low-energy photons) that would
otherwise give rise to high surface doses without contributing therapeutic dose at the target distance. Generally, only photons
(gamma rays or characteristic x rays) with energies >15 keV contribute therapeutically significant dose over the 3 to 50 mm range
of distances relevant to brachytherapy. However, this classical definition of a brachytherapy source (*i.e.*, radioactive material permanently sealed in a metal container), is rapidly becoming too narrow.
Balloon applicators inflated with radioactive solutions have been
proposed as a method for treating both malignant and benign proliferative processes (Dempsey *et al.*, 1998). Arterial stents, coated
with beta-emitting radionuclides, have been developed for prophy-
lactic treatment of cardiac arteries to prevent restenosis following
percutaneous angioplasty (Amols *et al.*, 1996b). A more general
and modern definition of a brachytherapy source would include any
device or applicator that physically confines activity within its
boundaries, delivers a therapeutic dose to nearby tissue, and
requires accurate positioning in the patient to deliver the prescribed dose to the intended target tissue.

The important physical properties of radionuclides commonly
used in brachytherapy are listed in Table 4.1. Table 4.2 lists the
radionuclides most commonly used for sealed source brachytherapy procedures classified according to the terminology described

TABLE 4.1—*Physical properties of brachytherapy radionuclides.*

Radionuclide	Half-Life	Photon Energy (MeV)	Half-Value Layer (mm Pb)	Exposure-Rate Constant[a] Γ_δ (R cm^2 mCi^{-1} h^{-1})	Physical Form
^{226}Ra[b]	1,600 y	0.83 (mean)	12	8.25[c]	Tubes, needles
^{222}Rn[b]	3.83 d	0.83 (mean)	12	8.25[c]	Seeds
^{60}Co	5.25 y	1.25 (mean)	12	13	Plaques, needles
^{137}Cs	30 y	0.662	6.5	3.2	Tubes, needles
^{192}Ir	74.02 d	0.397 (mean)	3	4.59	Seeds in ribbons, wires, source on cable
^{125}I	60.14 d	0.028	0.025	1.45	Seeds
^{103}Pd	17 d	0.020	0.008	0.86	Seeds
^{198}Au	2.7 d	0.412	3.3	2.35	Seeds
^{90}Sr/^{90}Y	28.2 y	2.24 (β max)	NA[d]	NA[d]	Plaques
^{241}Am	432 y	0.60	0.12	3.14	Tubes
^{169}Yb	32 d	0.093 (mean)	0.48	3.27	Seeds
^{131}Cs	9.69 d	0.030	0.030	1.24	Seeds
^{145}Sm	340 d	0.043	0.060	0.885	Seeds

[a]This subscript notation, δ, in Γ_δ is used to denote that the calculated value does not include the contributions of radiations removed (*i.e.*, attenuated due to the presence of encapsulating material).
[b]Listed for historical significance only.
[c]0.5 mm platinum-iridium filtration.
[d]NA = Not applicable.

TABLE 4.2—*Radionuclides used for implantation.*

Technique	Traditional	Current	Future
Intracavitary and Intraluminal Applications			
Low dose rate	^{226}Ra	^{137}Cs	^{241}Am, ^{192}Ir, ^{169}Yb
High dose rate	^{60}Co	^{60}Co, ^{192}Ir	^{192}Ir, ^{169}Yb
Interstitial Implants			
Preloaded	^{226}Ra	^{137}Cs	—
Afterloaded	—	^{192}Ir	^{125}I, ^{103}Pd, ^{169}Yb
High dose rate	—	^{192}Ir	^{192}Ir, ^{169}Y
Permanent Implants			
Conventional dose rate	^{222}Rn	^{198}Au	^{198}Au, ^{131}Cs
Ultra-low dose rate	—	^{125}I, ^{103}Pd	^{125}I, ^{103}Pd

previously. Properties such as half-life, photon energy, radiation output per unit activity, specific activity (Bq g^{-1}, Ci g^{-1}), fabrication cost, and toxicity all play a critical role in determining the clinical applications appropriate for each radionuclide. Because the three-dimensional dose-distribution characteristic of a given source is so important to appropriate clinical use, a short review of brachytherapy dosimetry principles is provided below.

4.2.1 *Specification of Source Strength for Photon Emitters*

The method of specifying strength of sealed radioactive sources strongly influences dose-calculation methodology and the level of dosimetric accuracy achievable. Historically, source strength has been specified by many different quantities and units including contained activity, apparent activity, equivalent mass of radium, mass of radium, and reference exposure rate. Unsealed radionuclides have historically been quantified in terms of true or contained activity. Despite frequent use of activity-based units, such as millicurie, curie and becquerel, sealed sources are almost never specified in terms of contained activity for the purposes of dose calculation or treatment prescription.

For purposes of radiation dosimetry, the term "kerma" relates to the kinetic energy liberated by uncharged particles; the energy expended to overcome binding energies, usually a relatively small component, is not included. Kerma (K) is the quotient of dE_{tr} by dm, where, dE_{tr} is the sum of the initial kinetic energies of all the changed particles in a mass dm of material, thus:

$$K = \frac{dE_{tr}}{dm}. \tag{4.1}$$

The unit of kerma is J kg^{-1} and the special name for the unit of kerma is the gray. The kerma rate $(\dot{K})$ is the quotient of dK by dt where dK is the increment of kerma in the time interval (dt). The unit of kerma rate is J kg^{-1} s^{-1} and the special name is gray per second (Gy s^{-1}) (ICRU, 1998a).

Sealed brachytherapy sources are calibrated and specified in terms of the radiation output (Gy h^{-1}) along the transverse bisector (*i.e.*, the axis perpendicular to and bisecting the long axis of the source). Specifically, source strength is specified in terms of air-kerma rate at a distance of 1 m from the source center. The measured result *shall* be corrected for scattering from surrounding surfaces (*e.g.*, walls, floors, etc.) as if a vacuum surrounded the source and detector. The resultant quantity, air-kerma strength, is defined as the product of the air-kerma rate in free space and the square of the distance and is denoted by the symbol S_K (Nath *et al.*, 1995). The units of air-kerma strength are μGy m^2 h^{-1} or cGy cm^2 h^{-1}, denoted in this Report by the symbol "U."[3] Units of cGy m^2 h^{-1} are often used in conjunction with high-intensity HDR sources.

$$1 \text{ U} = 1 \text{ } \mu\text{Gy m}^2 \text{ h}^{-1} = 1 \text{ cGy cm}^2 \text{ h}^{-1} = 10^{-4} \text{ cGy m}^2 \text{ h}^{-1}. \tag{4.2}$$

A number of older quantities remain in use (Williamson, 1991a). Cesium-137 tubes, ^{192}Ir seeds, and other radium substitutes are frequently specified in terms of the equivalent mass of radium with units of mgRaEq. The strength of a given source in mgRaEq is the mass (in milligrams) of ^{226}Ra, encapsulated in 0.5 mm of platinum-iridium that gives the same transverse-axis radiation output, or air-kerma strength, as the source. One mgRaEq source of ^{137}Cs or ^{192}Ir has an air-kerma strength (S_K) of 7.23 cGy cm^2 h^{-1}. Equivalent mass of radium simply describes the radiation output of a

---

[3]This should not be confused with the quantity "U" (use factor) commonly used in shielding calculations (see Glossary and Symbols and Acronyms).

source as a multiple of that of a 1 mg ^{226}Ra needle. Apparent activity, usually expressed in units of millicurie, is the air-kerma strength of a source relative to the output of a hypothetical 1 mCi point source consisting of the same radionuclide as the given source. Historically, apparent activity was used to quantify strength of permanently implanted sources such as ^{125}I and ^{198}Au. However, with newer developments in brachytherapy (e.g., ^{125}I liquid filled reservoir for treating cystic brain tumors) radioactive sources are frequently prescribed and assayed in activity units.

Use of air-kerma strength (or its numerically identical European counterpart, reference air-kerma rate) in clinical practice has been endorsed by various standards groups (Williamson et al., 1993). The radiation-oncology community is gradually replacing older units and quantities with air-kerma strength in areas of clinical practice. The quantity air-kerma strength should be used for specifying source strength in treatment planning and treatment prescription. NIST maintains primary S_K standards for the most commonly used LDR brachytherapy sources (Hanson, 1995). Transfer of these standards to individual clinical practices and source vendors is achieved by a network of secondary laboratories, known as Accredited Dosimetry Calibration Laboratories (ADCL) that are accredited and overseen by AAPM. For some sources, including HDR ^{192}Ir sources, ADCL maintains secondary standards based upon NIST's external-beam air-kerma standards. All clinical brachytherapy sources shall have source strength calibrations that are directly traceable to the primary or secondary air-kerma strength standards maintained by NIST or ADCL when such standards exist. Creation of an appropriate primary or secondary air-kerma strength standard should be considered as an essential component of developing and clinically implementing new photon-emitting brachytherapy sources (Williamson et al., 1998).

4.2.2 Determination of Absorbed Dose

In brachytherapy, computation and display of the dose distribution within and around the implanted volume is an essential element of current practice standards. The process of calculating the dose distribution for a patient implant is designated "treatment planning" and usually relies on digital computers equipped with specialized treatment planning software. The mathematical model used to calculate absorbed-dose rate, given the source locations, strengths, internal construction, and radionuclide is called the "dose-calculation algorithm."

Because direct measurement of absorbed dose near brachyther-apy sources is technically difficult, historical dose calculation algo-rithms have been based on semi-empirical models. The most widely used of these models is the isotropic point-source model described by the following equation:

$$\dot{D}_r = S_K \left(\frac{\mu_{en}}{\rho}\right)_{air}^{med} \frac{T_r}{r^2},$$
(4.3)

where:

$\dot{D}_r$ = absorbed-dose rate (in cGy h[-1]) in a medium at a distance r (in centimeters) from the point source

$\left(\dfrac{\mu_{en}}{\rho}\right)_{air}^{med}$ = mass-energy absorption coefficient ratio used to convert air kerma to absorbed dose in the medium surrounding the source.[4]

The factor, T_r is the ratio of the air kerma in the medium to that in air at distance r from the source. It describes the effect of the surrounding medium on absorbed-dose distribution and reflects the competition between attenuation of primary photons and buildup of scattered photons in the medium. For radium substitute radio-nuclides, T_r is approximately equal to one for distances up to 5 cm. The inverse square relationship, represented by the $1/r^2$ term, dom-inates the absorbed-dose distribution. This simple one-dimensional model is almost universally used for interstitial seed sources emit-ting photons with energies >300 keV. This model was first general-ized to extended sources (e.g., ^{137}Cs intracavitary tubes and needles) by Rolf Sievert in 1921 (Sievert, 1921). Reviews of this model show that it accurately models ^{137}Cs-source absorbed-dose distributions but cannot be assumed to accurately predict absorbed dose around lower energy sources (Williamson, 1996).

The simple analytic model described above is not sufficiently accurate for clinical use in the 60 to 100 keV energy range or in the 20 to 40 keV energy range of typical permanent implant sources. Inaccurate dosimetry has been a serious barrier to accu-mulation of consistent clinical experience with ^{125}I permanent implantation; the best estimate of the dose rate per apparent millicurie at 1 cm has changed since its introduction in 1964 (Williamson, 1991b). In the last decade, low-energy brachytherapy dosimetry has been placed on a firm foundation by validation and

---

[4]For a more complete discussion on the relation between exposure and various dose quantities, see Appendix A.1.

acceptance of two quantitative dosimetry methods: use of thermoluminescent dosimeters and Monte-Carlo photon-transport (MCPT) dosimetry calculations (Williamson, 1988; 1995; 1998). The former method consists of placing thermoluminescent dosimeters, along with the brachytherapy source, into precisely machined slots in a water-equivalent solid phantom. A multi-institutional, National Cancer Institute sponsored research contract on low-energy seed dosimetry demonstrated that low-energy source dose-rate distributions could be reproducibly measured with a precision of ±6 % (Anderson et al., 1990). This result encouraged clinical acceptance of measured dose-rate distributions and stimulated further research in this area. In contrast, MCPT simulation requires a rigorous numerical solution of the Boltzmann transport equation, which fully characterizes the absorbed-dose distribution in complex systems of sources and applicators. Comparison of MCPT calculations and thermoluminescent dosimeter measurements showed excellent agreement (i.e., within 2 to 3 %, between the two approaches) (Williamson, 1991b; 1994).

In order to facilitate clinical use of measured dose-rate distributions or those distributions derived from Monte-Carlo simulations, AAPM (Nath et al., 1995) endorsed a new dose calculation formalism specifically designed to use a sparse matrix of Monte Carlo or measured dose rates as its input in contrast to the classical semi-empirical models described by Equation 4.3. The formalism uses tables of dosimetric ratios to account for various effects (e.g., radial dose functions to account for dose falloff along the transverse axis and anisotropy functions to account for polar anisotropy). The report of AAPM (Nath et al., 1995) recommends a critically reviewed set of dosimetric parameters for two-dimensional dose-distribution data for several models of ^{125}I, ^{192}Ir, and ^{103}Pd seeds. Various authors have published dose-rate distributions for other sources using the format discussed in the report of AAPM (Das et al., 1997; Williamson and Li, 1995). The semi-empirical dose models and the AAPM calculations are in close agreement for ^{192}Ir and other radium substitutes but these models differ by as much as 15 % for ^{125}I interstitial seeds.

Generalizations of the classical isotropic source models using sievert methodology applied to the dosimetry of ^{137}Cs tubes are also sufficiently accurate for treatment planning purposes. For sources having average photon energies <300 keV, transverse-axis dosimetry *should* be based on carefully reviewed dose measurements or Monte-Carlo simulations. In this energy range, classical models *should not* be used for clinical dosimetry unless verified by Monte-Carlo or experimental dose-estimation techniques.

4.2.3 *Physical and Dosimetric Properties of Brachytherapy Sources*

Some of the important properties of photon-emitting brachytherapy sources include photon energy and abundance, half-life, specific activity, cost of production, toxicity and safety of the radionuclide and its decay products. Photon energy is less important in brachytherapy than in ERT. For sources emitting photons with energies >100 keV, the inverse square law predicts transverse-axis dose falloff within 5 % over the therapeutically significant distance range from 0 to 5 cm (Williamson, 1998). Only for very-low-energy sources (*e.g.*, ^{103}Pd and ^{125}I) does the depth-dose curve significantly deviate from the inverse square law. Moreover, absolute dose rate, as well as relative dose, is independent of the radionuclide and composition of the surrounding medium for sources emitting photons >200 keV (Williamson, 1998). This energy range includes all of the reactor-produced radium substitute materials widely used today in clinical brachytherapy. Low-energy photon sources, such as ^{125}I and ^{103}Pd, produce dose-rate distributions that significantly deviate from inverse square-law approximations, depend significantly on the atomic composition of the surrounding tissue, and are sensitive to small changes in photon spectrum. Even though penetration in tissue is essentially independent of photon energy >100 keV, the half-value layer in lead rises steeply with energy. Because they have nearly identical depth-dose characteristics, artificial brachytherapy radionuclides with mean photon energies >100 keV are often referred to as "radium substitutes."

4.2.4 *Sources for Low Dose-Rate Intracavitary Brachytherapy*

Intracavitary therapy sources come in a variety of shapes and sizes, are usually costly to fabricate, and may be used to treat target tissue 2 to 5 cm from the applicator (Figure 4.1). The use of long-lived radionuclides requires permanent encapsulation in a nontoxic metal such as stainless steel or platinum. These sources have approximate physical lengths from 20 to 25 mm, diameters from 2 to 3 mm, and active lengths from 13 to 15 mm. They become a part of an institution's radionuclide inventory and will be used to treat many patients over their useful half-life times. Tissue attenuation is one of the factors that limits the dose that can be delivered to the periphery of the target volume. Radium-226, with its very long half-life, was used for intracavitary treatment in the early 1900s, less than a decade after being isolated by Madame Curie. The clinical use of radium has almost disappeared because of safety hazards associated with the high-energy photons emitted by its daughter products as well as the gaseous physical state of its immediate daughter product, ^{222}Rn. Almost all modern LDR intracavitary brachytherapy treatment is performed using ^{137}Cs, a fission byproduct with a 30 y half-life. Its single gamma ray of 0.66 MeV is less penetrating than the 0.8 MeV (average energy) photons from radium and its decay products or the photons from ^{60}Co (Tables 4.1 and 4.2). Cesium-137 has solid decay products and is normally distributed as insoluble glass microspheres encapsulated in 0.5 to1.0 mm thick stainless steel. These sources produce far less hazard in the rare circumstance of a ruptured source than radium tubes but have dose distributions nearly identical to that of ^{226}Ra.

Originally, 1 Ci of activity was defined in terms of the rate of disintegration from one gram of ^{226}Ra. This led to the widespread practice of specifying source loadings in terms of the milligrams of ^{226}Ra contained within the sources. Because all radium-substitute radionuclides would have the same dose-rate constant, use of mgRaEq units meant that ^{226}Ra-loading rules could be applied unchanged to implants using ^{137}Cs or ^{192}Ir. In LDR brachytherapy, the product of source strength and treatment time was given in units of milligrams radium equivalent-hours (mgRaEq h). This term was widely used to prescribe or describe intracavitary treatments. The quantity corresponding to the product of S_K and treatment time in hours is referred to as the integrated reference air kerma (*IRAK*) with units of μGy m^2 (Williamson, 1993). Hence, 1 mgRaEq h = 7.23 Gy cm^2. In terms of these quantities, intracavitary sources have strengths ranging from 36 to 200 U, while the total air-kerma strength loaded into LDR intracavitary applicators ranges from 130 to nearly 1,500 U. The *IRAK* per patient treatment ranges from 80 to 400 Gy cm^2. Treatment times vary from 18 to 75 h.

Virtually any surgically accessible body site with a well-defined target volume can be treated with localized interstitial brachytherapy. Common sites for the use of this technique include localized tumors of the breast, head and neck, gynecological and genitourinary systems, extremities, brain and various body lumina including esophagus, biliary duct system and bronchi. Classically, platinum-iridium clad ^{226}Ra needles were implanted directly into the target tissue. Cesium-137 needles replaced the use of radium sources in the 1970s. Preloaded implant techniques expose all surgical-suite personnel to ionizing radiation and can result in the delivery of very high doses to the hands of the radiation oncologist. For this reason, interstitial implantation of radium and radium substitutes fell into disuse with the emergence of megavoltage external-beam treatment machines.

Interstitial brachytherapy experienced a renaissance in the 1960s when afterloading techniques using ^{192}Ir sources were introduced (Henschke et al., 1963; Pierquin, 1987). Iridium-192, with a 74 d half-life and an average photon energy of 0.4 MeV, is a widely used source for temporary interstitial implants. Although its average energy is significantly lower than that of [226]Ra, it produces radium-equivalent absorbed-dose distributions in tissue and can be cost-effectively generated in nuclear reactors to very high specific activities. In Europe, ^{192}Ir is often used in the form of a wire containing an iridium-platinum radioactive core encased in a sheath of platinum. In the United States, ^{192}Ir is available in the form of seeds (typically 0.5 mm in diameter by 3 mm long) with air-kerma strengths of 1 to 72 cGy cm^2 h^{-1}. The seeds are encapsulated in a 0.5 mm diameter nylon ribbon and are usually spaced at 1 cm center-to-center intervals. In addition to eliminating radiation exposure hazards in the operating room, ^{192}Ir ribbons and wires can be trimmed to the appropriate active length for each catheter. Typical loadings for interstitial implants range from 70 to 700 U with treatment times from 24 to 168 h, and *IRAK* values from 50 to 250 Gy cm^2. High specific activity ^{125}I seeds are also used for temporary interstitial implants. These sources are available in strengths from 5 to 50 U. Although these sources are not dosimetrically equivalent to radium substitutes and present more biological and dosimetric complexities than higher-energy sources, they have several advantages. Because of the low-energy photons emitted by ^{125}I, a thin lead-foil shield or even tissue overlying the implant site reduces ambient exposure rates dramatically, eliminating or reducing potential radiation hazards to the attending hospital staff or members of the public. In addition, thin high atomic number foils may be used to internally shield critical structures near the implant site. The most common temporary implant techniques are the use of ^{125}I seeds for episcleral plaque-therapy for intraocular melanoma, for retinoblastinoma, and for stereotactically guided brain implants. The thin (0.05 mm thick) titanium capsule wall of ^{125}I seeds can be ruptured by manual manipulation and handling, potentially releasing radioiodine into the environment. All thinly encapsulated high activity interstitial sources containing activity in a volatile form *should* be leak tested prior to each use in a patient.

4.2.5 *Sources for Permanent Interstitial Brachytherapy*

For permanent implants, minimizing radiation exposure to the general public has greatly influenced the choice of radionuclide.

Classically, high-energy radionuclides with half-lives on the order of a few days were used. Radon-222 gas encapsulated in gold tubing and later [198]Au seeds were used for permanent implants. The patient had to be confined to a controlled area until source decay reduced ambient exposures to acceptable levels. Such implants used initial prescription dose rates of 0.7 to 1 Gy h^{-1} and delivered most of the dose within one week, making them radiobiologically similar to LDR temporary implants. Classical permanent implantation techniques with [222]Rn or [198]Au delivered high doses to the radiation oncologist's hands and exposed inpatient hospital personnel to high-energy radiation.

Currently, longer-lived but very-low-energy photon emitters are used for permanent implantation (*i.e.*, ^{125}I and [103]Pd). A patient's own tissues or a thin lead foil are sufficient to limit exposure rates to very-low levels. Use of these sources reduces exposure to the radiation oncologist's hands and fingers and eliminates the need to hospitalize patients solely for radiation protection purposes. The low initial-prescription dose rates characteristic of low-energy seed implants, typically 0.03 to 0.2 Gy h^{-1}, require delivery of doses ranging from 100 to 145 Gy for definitive treatment as compared to doses between 60 to 80 Gy for classical LDR implants. Such implants are often described as "ultralow" dose rate. The most common use of such sources has been for permanent implantation in transperineal implantation of the prostate using transrectal ultrasound imaging to guide seed placement (Blasko *et al.*, 1987). These procedures involve the use of 50 to 200 seeds with source strengths from 0.4 to 3 U in order to achieve a minimum prescribed dose up to 145 Gy for ^{125}I seeds or up to 135 Gy for [103]Pd seeds as calculated according to AAPM (Nath *et al.*, 1995) recommendations.

4.2.6 *Sources for High Dose-Rate Brachytherapy*

Specific activity is an important source-selection criterion for HDR brachytherapy as well as for highly miniaturized LDR interstitial sources. Because of practical and theoretical limits on how much ^{137}Cs or [226]Ra can be concentrated into a small pellet, these radionuclides are not useful for HDR brachytherapy. Iridium-192 or ^{60}Co, both of which have precursors with large neutron capture cross sections and which can be produced with very high specific activities, are the radionuclides commonly used for HDR brachytherapy. More detailed discussion of these sources will be found in Section 4.3.4.

4.2.7 Beta-Ray Applicators and Eye Plaques

Strontium-90 in the form of a sealed source may be used to treat shallow lesions such as pterygium of the eye (Paryani et al., 1994). Strontium-90 is a fission product, which decays to ^{90}Y with a half-life of 28.9 y, which in turn decays to stable ^{90}Zr with a 64 h half-life. The most common applicator is in the form of a handheld plaque used to treat benign proliferative diseases of the eye. Surface dose rates of ~1 Gy s^{-1} can be produced with 1.85 to 3.70 GBq (50 to 100 mCi) plaques. Some techniques for regional therapy are discussed in Section 3.

The use of plaques containing radioactive materials for temporary implants has been adapted for treatment of tumors of the eye (e.g., retinoblastoma, choroidal melanoma, orbital rhabdomyosarcoma, and ocular metastases from other cancers). The plaque is sewn to the sclera, left in place for a calculated period of time and then removed. The first radionuclide employed for this technique was ^{60}Co (Buys et al., 1983). Due to the high-energy emissions from ^{60}Co, placement of the plaque in close proximity to the optic nerve had the potential to cause radiation-induced nerve damage. The use of plaques with lower energy sources, chiefly ^{125}I, reduced or eliminated these complications and gave favorable clinical results (Abramson et al., 1997; Melia et al., 2001). The lower energy plaques also offered radiation safety advantages (Myers and Abramson, 1988). More recently, plaques incorporating ^{106}Ru have found clinical acceptance and have been used in selected institutions for treatment of choroidal melanoma and other diseases of the eye (Georgopoulos et al., 2003; Murthy et al., 2005b).

4.2.8 Experimental Brachytherapy Sources

A number of radionuclides that emit low-energy photons in the 40 to 100 keV range have been considered and investigated for use in sealed-source brachytherapy. These include ^{169}Yb, ^{241}Am, and ^{145}Sm (Table 4.1) (Fairchild et al., 1987; ICRU, 2004; Mason et al., 1992; Perera et al., 1994; Piermattei et al., 1992). The use of ^{131}Cs sealed sources for interstitial implantation in cancer therapy was recently approved by FDA. In this photon energy range (4 to 34 keV), sources give rise to depth doses in tissue that are qualitatively similar to those of more conventional radium-substitute radionuclides and, therefore, closely approximate inverse square-law falloff. In contrast, ^{103}Pd and ^{125}I sealed sources with ultra-low photon energies (20 and 28 keV, respectively) have depth-dose characteristics significantly less penetrating than those predicted by inverse square-law models as discussed previously. The photons emitted by ^{169}Yb and ^{241}Am sources, averaging 93 and 60 keV, respectively, interact in water predominantly by elastic Compton interactions, giving rise to multiply-scattered photons that compensate for attenuation of the primary photons. However, unlike photons emitted from higher-energy radionuclides, low-energy photons interact by the photoelectric effect in lead and other shielding materials, offering the prospect of effectively shielding critical structures using individually-customized shields with thin metallic foils, typically made of gold or platinum-iridium of 0.5 mm thickness.

The use of ^{145}Sm (x-ray energy of 43 keV) interstitial seeds, encapsulated in titanium and having the same physical dimensions as commercially-available ^{126}I seeds, has been developed as mentioned above (Fairchild et al., 1987). In addition to the advantages of improved radiation protection and flexible internal shielding design, investigators have proposed using ^{145}Sm seeds to treat tumors that selectively incorporate iodine-bearing thymidine analogs into their deoxyribonucleic acid (Fairchild et al., 1982). Samarium-145 emits photons just over the K-absorption edge of iodine (33.2 keV) and releases an Auger electron cascade resulting in a highly localized dose of moderately elevated linear energy transfer (LET) radiation to the nuclei of tumor cells containing iodine.

4.3 Treatment Delivery Technology

This Section presents an overview of some of the technology used in applying brachytherapy techniques to various implant sites. However, this Report cannot present an exhaustive discussion of brachytherapy techniques. In particular, this Section is intended to emphasize the radiation safety issues associated with brachytherapy.

4.3.1 Permanent Implants

Permanent implants with either ^{198}Au, ^{125}I, or ^{103}Pd seeds can be performed in any surgically accessible body site. Tumor sites that have been implanted include brain (meningiomas), lung, recurrent head and neck cancer, retroperitoneal lymph nodes, and prostate. Historically, implantation required surgical exposure of the target area. Preoperative imaging and clinical examination are used to estimate the target-volume dimensions and the number and strength of radioactive seeds needed to deliver the prescribed dose. After surgically exposing the tumor, its dimensions are measured directly and the proposed implant design reevaluated. Manual calculation aids such as nomograms have been used to quickly determine the seed spacings required (Anderson et al., 1993). Various types of single-seed implantation instruments, such as the Mick Applicator® (Mick Radio-Nuclear Instruments, Inc., Mount Vernon, New York), can be used to implant seeds one-by-one. Typically, preloaded cartridges containing from 10 to 15 seeds are placed in the applicator. By ejecting each seed at a controlled distance, a linear array of seeds can be approximated. Seeds can also be placed using absorbable suture material containing from 5 to 10 seeds spaced at 1 cm intervals. These can be sutured directly to the exposed tumor bed or sutured to a gel-foam sheet in an array that is then sutured to the tumor bed. Linear arrays of seeds contained within a semi-rigid absorbable suture material are also available. The major radiation safety issues encountered with the use of these seeds include minimizing exposure to the operator's hands, inventory control, and minimizing large dose-delivery errors.

The most common permanent implant procedure is the transperineal prostate implant using transrectal ultrasound guidance (Blasko et al., 1987; Holm et al., 1983). A template with a rectangular array of holes is used to guide the perineal implant needles. The template may be rigidly mounted to the ultrasound probe. Usually, a pretreatment ultrasound examination, or "volume" study, of the patient in the treatment position has been performed. The transverse images are contoured to form a three-dimensional model of the target volume, anterior rectal wall, and urethra. These data are then downloaded into a treatment-planning computer. Treatment planning is used to optimize the needle locations, depths and loading sequence of radioactive seeds and spacers needed to achieve acceptable dosimetric coverage of the prostate and normal tissue sparing. On the day of treatment, the patient is immobilized and the volume study repeated. Under ultrasound guidance, the needles are positioned in as close an approximation as possible to the preoperative treatment plan. Following completion of the procedure, CT imaging is used to localize the seeds and delineate the prostate. The dose distribution is then recalculated to evaluate the technical success of the procedure. Transrectal ultrasound guided perineal implant procedures require meticulous attention to QA and accuracy of treatment planning and delivery to avoid large dose-delivery errors.

4.3.2 *Manual Afterloading*

Manually afterloaded intracavitary applicators were introduced into clinical practice in the early 1960s. The techniques for manual afterloading were first used as a replacement for radium-loaded applicators in gynecological applications. The more common applicators use a central intrauterine tandem and two vaginal colpostats positioned within the vagina. The vaginal colpostats may contain bladder and rectal shields with 3 to 5 mm thick tungsten alloy in the medial aspects of their anterior and posterior surfaces. The applicators are equipped with source holders for inserting tube sources or identical size dummy sources. A sequence (typically from two to six) of intracavitary sources can be loaded in tandem into the intrauterine region by means of a thin flexible plastic tube. To avoid exposure hazards, dummy sources are afterloaded into the applicators to permit radiographic examination of the implant. After the patient has been returned to her room, the prescribed radioactive sources are manually afterloaded into the applicator using handheld forceps and other tools for manipulating the sources.

Afterloading techniques can also be used for accessible body sites where catheters can be placed. Such sites include single nodes, brain cancers, head and neck cancers, and limbs. In the operating room, large trocar needles are used to implant flexible nylon catheters that will later hold ^{192}Ir ribbons. Typically, the patient remains hospitalized for 3 to 5 d after the operative procedure and before implantation to allow for wound healing. "Dummy" (*i.e.*, nonradioactive) ribbons are used to determine the location and length of ribbon to be inserted in each catheter and the dummy ribbons remain in place until imaging of the implant is complete. The dummy seeds are removed and the ^{192}Ir seeds in ribbons are then prepared. The patient is transported to his or her room and the ^{192}Ir ribbons are manually inserted. The ribbons are held in place by placing small metal buttons over the ends of the catheters and crimping these in place. Alternatively, the ends of each catheter can be heat sealed. Procedures can use either "double ended" flexible catheters, that require fixation at both the distal and proximal skin surfaces, or a variety of single-ended (often called "blind-ended") applicators, requiring fixation only at the proximal skin surface. Materials used include rigid steel needles as well as flexible plastic catheters. Manually afterloaded ^{192}Ir ribbons can be adapted for use in fixed-source train (Figure 4.1) or multiple-channel remote afterloading devices (Grigsby, 1992; Porter *et al.*, 1988).

4.3.3 *Low Dose-Rate Brachytherapy Remote*
Afterloading Systems

Remote afterloading systems robotically transfer sources from a
shielded storage container (or safe) to applicators in the patient
(Glasgow, 1993; 1995a). The device is connected to patient applicators *via* transfer tubes and transports sources either by means of
stepping-motor driven cables or compressed air. These devices are
controlled by a separate control panel located near but outside
the room door. This location allows nurses to retract the sources
before entering the room to render care and to resume treatment
after completing each nursing intervention. The devices then display the remaining treatment time along with the status of the
machine. Generally, an LDR remote afterloader automatically
retracts the sources after the programmed cumulative treatment
time has elapsed. Conventional remote afterloading systems utilize
multiple sources that are simultaneously transported to each
applicator and remain continuously in their treatment positions
unless the treatment is interrupted. The source strength and radionuclide loaded into the patient, the total treatment time prescribed, and total *IRAK* delivered are identical to a corresponding
manually afterloaded treatment. Any room in a facility that is designated as adequate by the RSO for treatment using LDR techniques should also be adequately shielded to accept an LDR remote
afterloader. Modifications will need to be made to accept the electronic controls and cabling for the afterloader. The device will also
need to be stored in a secure area when not in use. This area can be
within the treatment room or in an adjacent space. The major radiation protection advantage of LDR remote afterloading is the
reduction of exposure to nursing and other inpatient personnel who
attend the patient.

The most common form of source used for LDR remotely afterloaded intracavitary implants is ^{137}Cs in the form of spherical pellets. Each applicator of the programmable source-train device
consists of fixed treatment positions, each of which can be occupied
by a spacer or radioactive source allowing the user to program any
desired sequence of nonradioactive and radioactive pellets. The
radioactive sources and spacers are stored in separate compart-
ments of the main safe. Through a system of mechanical valves,
user-programmed sequences are assembled (composed) and placed
in the intermediate safe compartment coupled to the corresponding
applicator. Compressed air is used to pneumatically transport
the assembled source trains from the intermediate safe to the
applicator and automatically return them to the intermediate safe

on completion of the programmed treatment time or when interrupted by an operator. This design has been adapted to HDR devices.

4.3.4 High Dose-Rate Brachytherapy Remote Afterloading Systems

High dose-rate (HDR) brachytherapy blends traditional intracavitary, interstitial and transluminal dose delivery strategies with external beam-like instantaneous dose rates, outpatient treatment orientation, and dose-time-fractionation philosophy. A common model of remote afterloader uses ^{192}Ir source. Programmable source-train machines, using multiple high-intensity ^{60}Co spheres, are also available for intracavitary HDR brachytherapy (Chenery et al., 1985). Because the instantaneous dose rate is large (as much as 450 Gy h^{-1} at 1 cm), carefully crafted safety and QA programs are essential. The outpatient character of HDR brachytherapy creates an additional safety hazard (i.e., all complex series of tasks must be completed in a single, short time period).

The latest generation of remote afterloaders are single-stepping source devices using high intensity ^{192}Ir sources ($S_K = 4 \times 10^4$ cGy cm^2 h^{-1}) (Glasgow et al., 1993; 1995a). A single source, available with external diameters from 0.6 to 1.1 mm and lengths from 4 to 12 mm is located at the end of a drive cable or wire which sequentially stops at each preprogrammed treatment position, or "dwell" position, for a programmed treatment or "dwell-time" from 1 s to several minutes depending on the application. These systems can inject the source cable into as many as 24 treatment channels that communicate by means of transfer tubes connecting each applicator to the appropriate channel port on the machine. Unlike conventional manually or remotely afterloaded implants, which simultaneously treat all active source positions, a single-stepping source afterloader treats one dwell position at a time, by sequentially transporting the source to each implanted catheter, treating the programmed positions in sequence, retracting the source into the machine, inserting it into the next applicator, and repeating the process.

Because HDR brachytherapy is an outpatient modality, patient convenience is enhanced and there is a potential to reduce costs by eliminating the need to hospitalize many patients. Radiation exposure to personnel is almost completely eliminated. Finally, HDR brachytherapy offers the ultimate in technical flexibility, as each dwell position can be placed anywhere along the catheter track and its dwell-time programmed individually. Treatment planning software capable of optimizing target-volume coverage or dose uniformity through automated manipulation of the dwell-time distribution is offered by all major vendors.

The increased complexity, compression of time for planning and treatment delivery processes and rapid delivery of high-dose fractions characteristic of HDR brachytherapy create opportunities for serious treatment delivery errors (Thomadsen *et al.*, 2003). This modality requires a well-organized procedure, a larger technical staff, and a more complex and comprehensive QA program (Appendix C).

4.3.5 *"Pulsed" Dose-Rate Remote Afterloading Systems*

The pulsed dose-rate (PDR) remote afterloader is a relatively recent device that combines the single-stepping source technology, characteristic of HDR brachytherapy, with conventional inpatient-based LDR brachytherapy (Williamson *et al.*, 1995). One commercially available device uses a single 37 GBq (1 Ci) ^{192}Ir source welded to the end of a transfer cable to sequentially treat each dwell position. This device simulates continuous LDR brachytherapy by automatically administering a sequence of "mini" HDR fractions, generally at hourly intervals such that the average hourly dose rate is the same as that of the corresponding manually afterloaded treatment. Such fractions are described as "pulses" and the interval between successive pulses, during which the source remains in its shielded safe, is the "quiescent" period. In all other respects, PDR brachytherapy is identical to LDR brachytherapy. Patients must be hospitalized during the procedure and dose prescriptions and total treatment times are unchanged. In contrast to conventional remote afterloading technology, PDR brachytherapy supports:

- improvement of implant quality through manipulation of individual dwell-times;
- improved flexibility in choosing prescription dose rates by varying the pulse width unlimited by either source decay or a finite source inventory; and
- reduction in the overall time for the implant by confining nursing interventions to the quiescent periods.

A PDR system uses a single moving source with an instantaneous tissue dose rate as high as 45 Gy h^{-1} at 1 cm. If a PDR afterloader malfunctions and fails to retract the source from the patient, serious patient injury and large staff exposures could result if the source is not rapidly brought under control. In contrast, with conventional LDR systems, a source retraction failure would result in continuing dose delivery. Finally, use of the PDR system greatly increases the complexity of machine acceptance testing and QA, as well as implementation of individual patient procedures.

4.4 Specific Precautions and Procedures

This Section discusses specific precautions and procedures necessary for each type of brachytherapy procedure. This Section is not a substitute for information developed by other voluntary and scientific organizations that address clinical or medical-physics issues in more detail. This discussion provides a general overview of the types of precautions and procedures necessary for good radiation safety practice and addresses broadly the general state of practice.

4.4.1 *Manual Afterloading*

Manually afterloaded sources *should* always be handled utilizing radiation safety precautions that minimize whole-body and extremity exposure. Remote handling devices (*e.g.*, long-handled forceps) *should* always be used. Shielded workstations *shall* be available for source preparation and calibration.

Prior to applicator insertion and source loading, patients *should* be thoroughly informed regarding the nature of the procedure, any anticipated acute symptoms or complications, and any procedures or restrictions they may be expected to follow in order to maintain the integrity of their implant. The patient *should* also be informed of any restrictions that may be necessary for the safety of staff, visitors and other patients. Patients *should* understand clearly any limitations on ambulation, number and types of visitors, and limits on visitation time. If by virtue of impaired mental or medical condition, compliance with these instructions cannot be expected, appropriate use of medication and intensive observation by nursing staff *should* be considered. In a rare circumstance, the radiation oncologist may need to consider whether alternative treatment would better suit the patient.

Before removing brachytherapy sources from the source preparation area, the destination, patient identifier and hospital room, the strength, number and type of sources removed *shall* be recorded. The inventory of remaining sources *should* be reviewed and checked for consistency with the number of sources possessed by the institution and other sources in use. The strength and identity of the sources *shall* be verified prior to loading sources into the patient. This can be achieved by visually checking source serial numbers or strength-specific color codes. Sources *shall* be transported from the preparation area to the patient room in a shielded container labeled with a "radioactive materials" label indicating the type, number and strength of sources being transported.

Before loading radioactive sources into a patient, the patient's identity *shall* be confirmed and matched for consistency with the written prescription by two independent means. A wristband bearing the information "radioactive precautions" *should* be placed on the patient. A minimum of two individuals *should* participate in the loading of radioactive sources. One person *should* be assigned the task of verifying the loading sequence against the written prescription. During the loading process, the prescription *shall* be available and the identity of each source or source train checked as it is loaded into the appropriate applicator or catheter. Sources remaining in the transport container *should* be counted and returned to the inventory. A logbook *should* be maintained of all sources taken out of and returned to the inventory.

After sources are loaded, the following actions or procedures *should* be in place:

1. The date and time of source insertion *shall* be documented on the prescription along with the anticipated date and time of source removal. Copies of the prescription *should* be placed on or within the patient's chart. The exterior of the patient's chart *should* be labeled with the standard radiation symbol and with the measured exposure rates. If the chart is electronic, provision *should* be made for information on radiation precautions to appear in some manner each time the chart is accessed during the period when the implant is in place.

2. The room *should* be posted with signs, "caution radioactive materials," as well as posted as a "radiation area." Also, information for visitors *should* be posted.

3. The exposure rate, air kerma rate, or dose rate *shall* be determined at a standard distance, such as 1 m from the approximate center of the implant in the patient with an appropriately calibrated survey meter, such as a portable ion chamber. When in the judgment of the RSO the use of portable shielding is deemed necessary, measurements at the doorway and in any surrounding areas protected by portable shields *should* be made and recorded in the radiation safety log, whether manually or electronically, to insure correct placement. The total exposures to medical

personnel or any unsupervised individuals, including visitors, over the life of the implant *should* be assessed for consistency with the facility's ALARA program.

4. Written orders pertaining to radiological and patient safety *shall* be available including special procedures (*e.g.*, closure or restriction of surrounding rooms) required to satisfy ALARA dose limits.

For each procedure, a method *should* be developed for medical personnel to check the integrity and position of the implant. Written nursing procedures, specific for the implant type, *should* be immediately available on the inpatient unit. These procedures *should* include emergency procedures, access control, and recognition of source positioning. Before 50 % of the dose is delivered, the manual or computer assisted calculations used to determine the treatment time and source loading needed to fulfill the written prescription *shall* be independently reviewed. The individual initially preparing the calculations and the reviewer *should* be a qualified medical physicist.

4.4.2 *Patient Care Precautions During Treatment*

Inpatient nursing staff *shall* control access to brachytherapy treatment rooms by healthcare personnel not involved in the treatment and by the public. Nursing personnel are responsible for ensuring compliance with restrictions defined in the patient's chart. Medical personnel *should* check the integrity of the implant at intervals specified by the responsible radiation oncologist.

A radiation oncologist or other physician with appropriate medical and radiation safety training *shall* be available on an on-call basis at all times while brachytherapy treatments are in progress. Also, a medical physicist or medical health physicist *should* be available. Nurses *shall* notify these individuals promptly in the event of missing or displaced sources, significant changes in implant position, or any other circumstance that may threaten the safety of personnel, the public, or the patient and may jeopardize the delivery of the planned dose. Procedures for dealing with dislodged sources *should* be part of the nursing manual. A shielded container and tools for the remote handling of a source, source train, or applicator containing sources *shall* remain in the patient's room for the duration of the implant. This container *should* be of sufficient size and shielding to safely hold any sources that could become accidentally dislodged. If the individual responsible for removing the sources fails to appear at the designated time, nursing personnel *shall* contact the responsible radiation oncologist or on-call physician. Modifications to the source loading or implant duration *should* be noted in writing on the written prescription including the copy posted in the patient's chart. Linens, food, utensils, trash and excreta are not contaminated. However, linens and trash *should* remain in the room until surveyed to ensure that no displaced sources are present. Any special circumstances *should* be clearly noted in the radiation-oncologist's orders or the procedure-specific nursing instructions in the nursing manual.

4.4.3 *Patient Care Precautions During Source Removal*

Surgical dressings and bandages near the implanted applicators or sources *shall* be removed carefully and checked by the radiation oncologist, or other appropriately trained medical staff, taking care not to dislodge the implant. Individuals responsible for changing such dressings *should* have training in source recognition, source-handling procedures, basic radiation safety procedures, and ability to assess correct implant position and integrity. Sources and applicators *shall* be removed by an appropriately trained individual, preferably the radiation oncologist. Any required pain medication *should* be ordered at a time sufficiently in advance of the unloading so that the procedure is not compromised. Sources *shall* be removed using a remote handling device and placed immediately into a shielded container. The date and time of source removal *shall* be documented on the prescription or treatment record and in the patient's chart. As the sources are being removed, the physician *shall* count the number of intracavitary sources or interstitial ribbons removed to verify that all sources documented on the written prescription have been removed.

After removal of the sources from the patient's room, a careful survey of the patient, the treatment room, and removed applicators *shall* be performed using an appropriate survey meter (*e.g.*, a GM detector) and the results documented in the treatment record, radiation safety log, and in the patient's chart. The treatment room *shall not* be released for cleaning and occupancy by another patient until:

- the sources are removed from the room and secured;
- the number of sources removed is reconciled with the number known to have been loaded; and
- the radiation survey verifies that no sources remain in the room.

The sources *should* be promptly returned to the source preparation area where a second source-by-source (seed-by-seed) count *should* be performed. Following this count, the sources *should* be returned to their permanent storage location, and the number of sources in that safe or storage receptacle checked for consistency with the relevant number of sources possessed by the institution, including those in use for other purposes. Cleaning or sterilization of surgical equipment *should* only be performed after a survey demonstrates that there is no residual activity. In the unusual circumstance that it becomes necessary to leave the sources in a patient room, the container *should* be made secure against unauthorized access or removal and properly labeled. In such circumstances, the nursing staff *shall* continue to treat the room as a restricted area. If a source appears to be lost, the responsible radiation oncologist, medical physicist and RSO *shall* be contacted immediately and the patient's room secured.

4.4.4 *Low Dose-Rate Remote Afterloading*

Within 24 h of initiating an LDR remotely afterloaded treatment, the correct operation of the system and its ancillary safety devices *shall* be confirmed by performing standardized daily QA tests (Appendix C). The individual programming the remote afterloader *shall* have available the written prescription or treatment plan defining the prescribed sequence of sources and treatment times in each channel.

Prior to initiating treatment, the setup and afterloading program *shall* be independently checked. The correct correspondence and connection of programmed channels and implanted applicators *should* be confirmed. This check of the initial programming and patient setup *should* be performed by a qualified medical physicist and radiation oncologist. During treatment, a radiation oncologist and a qualified medical physicist *should* be available on-call at all times. The qualified medical physicist *should* be skilled in afterloader operation and management of emergency or malfunction conditions.

As the treatment room is entered, the sources *shall* automatically retract. This withdrawal will result from the interruption of an interlock switch located on the treatment room door. The room *shall* also be provided with an area monitor that will indicate the presence or absence of radiation to persons entering the treatment room. To avoid prolonging the treatment, interruptions and visits to the patient *should* be minimized. Whenever the treatment is interrupted, the treatment room door *shall* remain open. To avoid unintentional irradiation of visitors and staff, operators *shall* visually confirm that the treatment room is occupied only by the patient before resuming treatment.

Should the area monitor or treatment device indicate a source retraction failure at the end of treatment or following an interruption command, the responsible medical physicist *shall* be informed immediately. Malfunctions of the afterloader or its ancillary safety systems *shall* be brought to the immediate attention of the on-call radiation oncologist and medical physicist.

Until the sources are brought under control, nursing staff *shall* practice appropriate manual afterloading safety precautions. Nursing staff and the responsible medical physicist *shall* follow documented emergency procedures. Staff *shall* be trained in emergency procedures during the initial installation of the device and at annual intervals thereafter. Following completion of treatment, a careful survey of the patient, the treatment room, removed applicators, and the afterloading housing *shall* be performed using a calibrated survey meter (*e.g.*, GM detector) to confirm complete retraction of the sources. The results *shall* be documented in the patient's treatment record. The treatment room *shall not* be released for cleaning and occupancy by another patient until the radiation survey is complete and is negative for incompletely retracted sources.

4.4.5 *High Dose-Rate Remote Afterloading*

High dose-rate (HDR) brachytherapy is typically performed as an outpatient procedure with daily dose fractions ranging from 2 to 10 Gy delivered in a few minutes using high intensity sources with instantaneous dose rates as high as 4.6×10^4 cGy cm^2 h^{-1}. The combination of large dose fractions, short time frames, intense pressure on personnel, enhanced technical flexibility, and complexity of treatment planning and delivery devices creates potential opportunities for treatment-delivery errors. Because of the high doses per treatment fraction and small number of fractions compared with typical ERT, recovery from errors is difficult and the consequences of error are potentially significant. A well-organized and well-trained treatment-delivery team (radiation oncologist, medical physicist, dosimetrist, and therapist) is essential. The need for detailed written procedures, checklists, written communication, and personnel training is especially critical in HDR brachytherapy. Various groups have developed comprehensive protocols for developing and maintaining safe treatment delivery processes (Kubo *et al.*, 1998; Kutcher *et al.*, 1994; Nath *et al.*, 1997).

4.4.5.1 *Organization of the Treatment Delivery.* At a minimum, there are four essential participants on the team: the radiation oncologist, the medical physicist, the dosimetrist, and the treatment unit operator, usually a radiation therapist. A successful program *shall* require a well-qualified and integrated treatment-delivery team with substantially more expertise than that afforded by formal certification processes. The additional expertise, required above and beyond board certification, is usually acquired through training by the device manufacturer, focused self-study, careful planning and preparation, extensive practice with the devices either onsite or at a participating facility, and visits to established HDR brachytherapy programs (Callan *et al.*, 1995).

Computerized treatment planning *shall* be available for HDR treatments. At a minimum, each institution providing HDR brachytherapy *shall* develop written treatment procedures defining:

- the step-by-step sequence by which the procedure is performed including the critical duties of each team member;
- information to be captured at each step and how it is to be recorded; and
- critical actions and decision points where a redundant QA check is needed.

4.4.5.2 *Documentation Requirements.* Accurate HDR treatment planning and delivery requires accurate information transfer among delivery team members working in the operating room, the simulator room, and the treatment-planning and -delivery areas. The radiation oncologist, medical physicist, dosimetrist, and therapist *should* cooperate closely and communicate accurately and unambiguously. All critical information, including applicator types used, relation of target volume to applicators, dose prescription, and simulator localization data *shall* be recorded on appropriate forms by individual team members primarily responsible for each corresponding activity. This form *should* accompany the patient chart and treatment folder as the patient proceeds through applicator insertion, treatment planning and treatment delivery. Each facility *should* develop forms for the following functions:

- written prescription and daily treatment record;
- daily remote afterloader QA protocol;
- physicist's treatment plan and documentation review; and
- documentation of implant geometry, simulation data, and verification of computerized dwell-time calculations.

No form is more critical to the safe execution of HDR brachytherapy than the treatment prescription and daily treatment record. This form functions as an overall summary of the multifraction course of therapy, including the current status of treatment (total dose and number of fractions given) and the written prescription. Manual or computer assisted calculations used to determine the dose delivered *should* be included in the patient's chart and separately in a treatment folder depending on the type of facility. The individual initially preparing the calculations or the reviewer *should* be a qualified medical physicist. More detailed descriptions of individual fractions (*e.g.*, dwell-time distributions) *should* be filed in separate sections of the chart. This form *should* be brief and general so that critical questions can be quickly answered.

Each facility *shall* develop a clearly defined prescription form documenting:

- fraction size;
- number of fractions;
- total dose;
- dose specification criteria;
- radiation oncologist's signature and date;
- location of the active dwell positions or applicator system relative to the written prescription;
- the identity of the applicator system; and
- the identity of the remote afterloader including some specific identification system if more than one unit is available.

The daily treatment record *shall* show the date and dose of each fraction delivered, the cumulative total dose, the source strength, total dwell-time, and applicator system used.

All detailed documentation specific to each fraction *should* be filed in a clearly marked section in the chart. All forms *shall* contain the patient's name and date of treatment. At a minimum, the chart and treatment folder *shall* include a detailed implant diagram, documenting the correspondence between catheter (channel) numbering system relative to external anatomy and radiographic images of each catheter, and also the graphic treatment plan (*e.g.*, isodose plots) or other calculations used as the basis of remote-afterloader programming.

4.4.5.3 *Treatment Specific Quality-Assurance Recommendations.* A detailed discussion of quality-assurance (QA) recommendations is beyond the scope of this Report. Recommendations on the type of

QA checks that may be performed are given in Appendix C and in the reports published by the American College of Radiology, the American Association of Physicists in Medicine, and the American College of Medical Physics. These recommendations are supplemental to the recommendations of the manufacturer and may be less specific than those procedures recommended by the professional organizations mentioned above.

In this Section, emphasis has been placed upon positional accuracy. A significant percentage of reported treatment delivery errors involve programming of incorrect positions into the treatment device that result in administration of treatment to the wrong site. This problem is due to the large number of variables (*e.g.*, calculation of dwell-times, entry of wrong activity or data, verification of patient identity) needed to support the increased positional flexibility of single-stepping source machines. The calculations needed to derive these parameters are simple but *shall* be verified (Ezzell, 1995). As most single-stepping source machines have no interlocks to prevent applicator-channel mismatches, only redundant manual checks can exclude delivery of dwell position sequences to the wrong applicator. When the dwell-time is derived from manual calculations, they *shall* be reviewed by a second individual not involved in the initial calculation. When the dwell-time is calculated by the treatment planning computer program, an independent manual- or computer-based (using different software and operator) calculation *shall* be performed. If the physicist performs the treatment planning, or works closely with a dosimetrist, a third person uninvolved in the original planning *should* review the dwell-time and source position calculations. The review process *should* be reviewed and signed by a qualified medical physicist (Neblett and Wesick, 1995; Van Dyke *et al.*, 1993). The qualified medical physicist *should* also review all treatment parameters, including data entry from radiographs or other imaging systems.

Upon completion of an HDR treatment or whenever treatment is interrupted, complete source retraction *shall* be confirmed both by means of the area monitor or by a handheld survey instrument. The survey instrument *should* be selected carefully so that the instrument does not saturate in high radiation fields. The selected instrument *shall* be checked for an appropriate response near the exposed HDR source well in advance of the patient treatment. If false readings in high-intensity fields could occur, an ion chamber survey meter *should* be used to cover the upper extreme of the exposure-rate range. Before each treatment the physicist's QA checks *shall* include checks of the functioning of radiation detectors.

4.5 High Dose-Rate Emergency Procedures and Treatment Attendance Requirements

Significant radiation injury could result from an HDR source becoming detached from its cable during treatment or if it failed to retract. Several investigations have focused on these issues (NRC, 1993a; 1993b; Thomadsen, 1995). Fortunately, the incidence of these dangerous events seems to be quite small and the failure of source retraction is considered highly unlikely. Despite the low probability of this event, all institutions practicing HDR brachytherapy *shall* develop appropriate emergency procedures for rapidly bringing an unretracted source under control and *shall* train staff in them. Such procedures *shall* also address emergency removal of the applicator system from the patient.

It *should* be assumed that a source retraction failure exists under any of the following conditions:

- the area monitor indicates a radiation field when the HDR system is interrupted;
- an error condition, as indicated by a code number consistent with source-retraction failure, appears on the console; and
- a portable survey meter indicates a radiation field during treatment-interrupt status.

Any of the above conditions *should* result in the following immediate emergency actions on the part of the physicist and the operator:

1. The physicist *should* interrupt the use of the HDR unit and activate the emergency retraction system available at the console.
2. The physicist *should* enter the room with a portable survey meter to verify the existence of a source retraction failure. If the source is not completely retracted, the physicist *should* activate the emergency retraction drive using the control system inside the treatment room.
3. If the survey indicates that radiation continues to be present, the physicist *should* manually retract the source.
4. If radiation is still present and the implant is designated "easily removable," the radiation oncologist *should* remove the applicators, secure them in the emergency shielded container, and verify that the patient is free of radioactive sources.
5. If the implant is not easily removable, the radiation oncologist *should* disconnect the transfer tubes from the

indexer, extract the source cable from the applicator, place the source cable intact into the shielded source holder, a so-called "bail out box" within the treatment room, and remove the patient from the room. If this procedure is not possible, the source *should* be moved away from the patient, the cable *should* be cut, and the distal cable fragment secured in a shielded storage container.

6. If radioactive material remains in the patient, the physicist and radiation oncologist *should* seal the proximal ends of the applicators, remove the applicators, and secure them in a shielded container.

These conditions require that the physicist and radiation oncologist carefully think through the process of applicator removal for all temporary implants including difficult interstitial implants (*e.g.*, base of tongue) and develop detailed written procedures for removing the catheters (Thomadsen, 1995). These emergency procedures *should* be practiced in dry runs at least once a year by all persons likely to be involved in patient treatment. The operator's manual *shall* be available at the console whenever patient treatment is performed. Some implant techniques, such as implantation of sites inaccessible for catheter removal except in an operating room, may not be suitable for HDR brachytherapy if they are overly complex or involve medically risky applicator removal techniques. Under no conditions *shall* open-ended applicators that allow a detached source to lodge interstitially in the patient's tissues be used for HDR brachytherapy.

A medical physicist and an individual qualified to remove the applicators from the patient under emergency conditions *shall* attend all treatments and *shall* be prepared to detect emergency conditions and implement the appropriate responses.

4.6 Addressable Events

In any use of brachytherapy techniques, there exists a potential for radiation injury. It is essential that any deviation from established techniques or procedures be addressed as rigorously as possible, whether a regulatory requirement or not. An addressable event may be considered to be any clinical or technical event that occurs in the course of planning, executing or managing a brachytherapy procedure that has a significant adverse effect on the safety or efficacy of the procedure and that could have been avoided by appropriate procedural changes.

The following are examples of addressable events:

- use of a radionuclide or source type in a therapeutic procedure other than the source or radionuclide prescribed;
- administration of a treatment or procedure to a patient other than the intended patient;
- administration of a therapeutic dose to an area other than the area prescribed;
- errors in computation, calibration, treatment time, source placement, source strength, or equipment malfunction such that the calculated total treatment dose delivered differs from the final prescribed dose by >20 %;
- failure to account for effects on dose distribution of prior, concurrent or subsequent radiation treatment, of medication(s), or of medical procedures that may compromise therapeutic efficacy; and
- delivery of a therapeutic treatment dose in a single fraction of a fractionated prescription such that the administered dose in the individual treatment differs from the dose prescribed for that individual treatment by >50 %.

The evaluation of an addressable event resulting from a brachytherapy procedure can be complex. A careful analysis of the cause or causes *should* be performed. Complexities arise due to difficulties in defining the treatment volume, specification of dose contours, and evaluation of the prescription itself. The causal analysis *should* address a review of the records of the procedure, review of policies and procedures, consideration of equipment performance, and training and education. The review team *should* be under the direction of an individual experienced in such analyses who was not involved in the procedure. The services of a qualified medical physicist *shall* be available in the evaluation of an addressable event. Services provided by the medical physicist *shall* include the evaluation of the actual dose delivered and an evaluation of the procedural systems in place. The medical physicist, radiation oncologist, and RSO *shall* develop a plan of action to prevent future occurrences. Remediation, including further education of personnel as appropriate or development of further safeguards *should* be implemented. It is essential that a thorough review of pertinent policies and procedures be performed to determine the cause of the event. Federal and local regulatory agencies will have specific requirements regarding the reporting of medical events. These regulations *should* be familiar to the RSO and the administration of the facility.

Addressable events involving brachytherapy *shall* be reported to the RSO and treating radiation oncologist as soon as these events are discovered. The RSO in consultation with the treating radiation oncologist and the administration of the facility can then determine if these events meet regulatory standards for reportability. These events *should* also be reported to the patient and the referring physician as soon as possible, preferably within one working day of the discovery. Doses *shall* be calculated to evaluate the doses to specific organs. The attending radiation oncologist *should* decide if there would be any expected medical consequences of an event, either short- or long-term. Appropriate interventions *shall* be considered in light of the patient's overall medical condition, the medical consequences of the event and the effects of any intervention. Short- and long-term medical management of such events *should* be planned carefully on an individual basis.

Even if an addressable event results in no demonstrable harm to the patient, it may represent a procedural lapse, a breakdown in existing systems, or lead to the identification of systematic problems that need to be addressed. Addressable events also may result from human error. However, such a finding *should* require consideration of factors that contribute to these errors, including the workload of the individual, staffing issues, and the working environment.

4.7 Readmission

When patients with permanent seed implants are admitted to an inpatient facility, written nursing procedures specific for the implant type *should* be immediately available on the inpatient unit. If a patient is being readmitted for medical reasons, the facility *should* develop a system whereby patients who still contain significant amounts of radioactive materials are recognized upon admission. The RSO *should* be notified in these circumstances and *should* provide instructions to staff and place radiation precautions in the chart as necessary. Depending on the site implanted, it is possible for seed(s) to be lost through urine, sputum or other body excreta. These losses may occur while the patient is in the hospital or after the patient is discharged. A common time when seeds may be lost is during removal of catheters or drains, especially Foley catheters. Clinical staff *should* be instructed in the recognition of the types of seeds used by the facility. Any suspected loss of seeds *should* be reported to the radiation safety staff and the responsible radiation oncologist.

4.7.1 *Inventory Control*

A common problem with permanent implants has been verification of the number of seeds used (Stutz *et al.*, 2003). Before seeds are used for implantation, a careful seed count *should* be performed and entered into the source inventory log maintained by the facility. To avoid problems with seed sterilization, some facilities are using prepackaged, sterile sources with a seed count verified by the manufacturer. As the implant procedure progresses, it *should* be possible for a member of the implant team (*e.g.*, a physicist, resident or therapist) to independently verify the seed count. A member of the surgical team *should* be assigned the task of counting seeds or seed arrays as they are used. Before the radiation-oncology team leaves the surgical area, the seed counts *should* be verified. If there is a discrepancy in the count, radiation safety staff *should* be notified and the room *should* be checked for any seeds that may be lost in the surgical area. These checks may be performed using portable survey meters, such as GM counters or sodium-iodide [NaI (Tl)] scintillation survey meters. If no seeds are found in the surgical area, it is possible that the count has not been kept correctly. Seeds not used *should* be promptly returned to the source preparation area where a seed-by-seed count *should* be performed to verify the seed count. If a CT scan is performed on the patient post-implant and predischarge, the CT scan may be used as a further verification of the seed count if a discrepancy still exists. The source custodian *should* record the number of seeds used and the number of seeds returned and verify the accuracy of the seed count.

4.7.2 *General Radiation Safety Procedures*

Following completion of the surgical procedure, whether on an inpatient or outpatient basis, a member of the implant team *shall* measure the radiation exposure from the patient on the surface of the patient's body and at 1 m from the approximate center of the implant. These measurements *shall* be made using a calibrated ionization chamber survey meter. These readings *shall* be entered into "radiation-precaution" tags placed in the patient's chart. The tags *shall* also indicate the date on which radiation precautions are no longer necessary. Because both ^{125}I and ^{103}Pd emit low-energy photons that are readily absorbed in tissue, the amount of overlying tissue will usually influence the exposure rate. A radiation survey of the operating room *shall* be performed by a member of the implant team using a sensitive survey meter (*e.g.*, a scintillation detector) to confirm that no radiation sources are left in the room or in materials from the procedure before room cleaning can be started.

Prior to release of either the inpatient or outpatient setting, the attending radiation oncologist, medical physicist or RSO *shall* provide the patient with radiation precautions appropriate to his individual circumstances. These instructions *shall* include the possibility of the loss of seeds, importance of maintaining distance, and special care with regard to minors. A record of this interview *should* be part of the radiation safety record. Prior to discharge, patients *should* be supplied with a document verifying the specifics of the implant as well as with information for contact with the department (Dauer *et al*., 2004; Smathers *et al*., 1999). The contact information *should* include a telephone number that will allow patients to call for response to any questions arising post-implant as well as a number for questions from authorities in the event that the presence of the patient activates radiation detectors installed in public access areas or transportation checkpoints.

4.8 Emergency/Off-Hours Response

A list of names and 24 h telephone numbers of individuals to contact in the event of a radiation emergency *shall* be available. This list is separate in function from listings of persons responding to radiation disasters or emergencies in emergency rooms or trauma centers. Personnel to be contacted may include the RSO and the responsible radiation oncologist or the radiation-oncology resident or fellow on-call. These lists *shall* be available to medical personnel caring for the patient. Specific instructions for emergency situations are given in Section 6.

4.9 Other Applications

This Section is intended to describe some new areas of development in brachytherapy sources and in the use of brachytherapy techniques.

4.9.1 *Intravascular Brachytherapy*

Percutaneous transluminal balloon angioplasty (PTA) is an important method of treating both peripheral and coronary artery disease in which case PTA is called percutaneous transluminal coronary angioplasty (PTCA). The primary complication following either PTCA or PTA is restenosis, a narrowing of the arterial lumen in response to injury inflicted on the vessel by the procedure required. Estimates of the incidence of clinically significant restenosis range from 20 to 50 %. Endovascular irradiation, administered immediately following the PTA procedure, was one of the few interventions that dramatically reduced the incidence of restenosis (Massulo *et al.*, 1996; Nath and Roberts, 1996; Schopohl *et al.*, 1996; Tierstein *et al.*, 1997).

Brachytherapy treatment systems fall into two major categories:

- stent-based therapy, in which an intracoronary stent which is itself radioactive or impregnated with radioactive material, is permanently placed at the PTCA site; and
- catheter-based therapy, in which a radioactive source is transported through a guide catheter and temporarily positioned at the treatment site until a prescribed dose is delivered.

Typical dose fraction sizes range from 10 to 20 Gy at the luminal surface or external elastic lamina. These distances are typically 2 to 3 mm from the catheter center for coronary arteries and as much as 5 mm from the catheter center for peripheral arteries.

A minimal treatment time reduces both cost and medical risk to the patient. Iridium-192 sources produce dose distributions that offer excellent coverage of the arterial wall without excessive dose to the endothelial layer, and the sources can be used in both cardiac and peripheral arteries. Iridium-192 sources are backed by the most extensive clinical and preclinical experience (Amols, 2002). It has been demonstrated that safe and effective treatment can be rendered using manually afterloaded ^{192}Ir ribbons with dose rates as high as 4,000 Gy m^2 h^{-1} (Tierstein *et al.*, 1997). However, the high level of activity needed to produce adequate dose rates carries the potential for significant personnel exposures. Limiting radiation exposure is important because catheterized patients cannot be moved to shielded vaults for treatment and because anesthesiologists and cardiologists will not leave the patient's side. For these reasons, conventional ^{192}Ir-based HDR brachytherapy units, unless available as a dedicated unit in a structurally shielded cardiac catheterization laboratory, are impractical (Bohan, 2000).

Radiation safety issues with any of these devices generally fall into three categories:

1. *Shielding of the treatment room*: Because these devices will most likely be used in rooms with shielding designed for diagnostic x-ray energies, an evaluation of the shielding and the dose rates in surrounding areas *shall* be performed

by a qualified medical physicist or qualified medical health physicist. This evaluation *should* consider the number of procedures possible without exceeding the permissible dose limits in surrounding areas. Portable shielding may be used to supplement the structural shielding. However, its location and use *should* be specified by the qualified medical physicist or qualified medical health physicist (Balter *et al.*, 2000; Bohan *et al.*, 2000; Folkerts *et al.*, 2002).

2. *Treatment of the correct anatomical location*: The correct positioning of the source relative to the area of restenosis is critical to effective treatment. Incorrect positioning of the source has been identified as a source of abnormal occurrences in the reports from regulatory agencies (NRC, 2004). The QA plan *shall*, therefore, consider the criteria for ensuring correct positioning and QA checks specific for positioning *shall* be performed within 24 h of the administration of treatment.

3. *Failure of the source to retract*: The failure of the sealed source to retract into its housing has been identified as a source of abnormal incidents with intravascular brachytherapy devices (NRC, 2004). Treatments with sealed sources *shall not* be undertaken without the presence of some type of "bailout box," a shielded container that can house the sealed source temporarily until a complete QC check of the intravascular brachytherapy device can be made. To avoid or minimize this situation, therefore, a check of the ability of the source to retract and emerge successfully *shall* be part of the QA procedures performed immediately prior to the treatment.

The development and successful use of drug-impregnated stents has made intravascular brachytherapy with radiation a limited technique. There may, however, remain a smaller group of patients (*e.g.*, patients with stenosis in peripheral veins in limbs) for whom radiation applications are the treatment of choice.

4.9.2 *Other Experimental Applications*

Various radionuclide sources have been proposed for intracavitary applications. Applicator systems have been successfully developed for ^{241}Am sources (Nath *et al.*, 1988, Samuels *et al.*, 1991). Small ^{169}Yb seeds have been used as replacements for ^{192}Ir for temporary interstitial implants (Piermattei *et al.*, 1995). Americium-241 has a low specific activity and high self-absorption which limits its use in LDR brachytherapy. Ytterbium-169 has a high specific activity (370 TBq mm^{-3}, ~10 Ci mm^{-3}) and it is possible that high-intensity ^{169}Yb sources could be used to deliver HDR intraoperative brachytherapy treatments in a lightly shielded operating room, potentially broadening the clinical applications of brachytherapy. The use of ^{169}Yb sources for permanent implantation is limited by the emission of 308 keV photons which increase the radiation protection hazards.

Californium-252, a radionuclide that emits fission neutrons with an average energy of 2.14 MeV, has been intensively investigated as a potential source for intracavitary treatment of gynecological neoplasms (Maruyama et al., 1997). Approximately 60 % of the absorbed dose arising from sealed ^{252}Cf sources is due to neutron emissions. One of the rationales for the use of ^{252}Cf is combining the advantages of conventional brachytherapy with the presumed benefits of high-LET therapy. This advantage is balanced by the increased radiation protection problems that arise due to the necessity for the use of combined photon and neutron shields, typically a combination of lead and a hydrogenous material such as polyethylene, to attenuate the radiation fields. Of equal importance is the increase in the relative biological effectiveness for neutrons as the dose rate decreases. The use of ^{252}Cf requires extreme caution and special attention from the RSO for the protection of personnel.

4.9.3   Use of High Dose-Rate Units for Intraoperative Radiation Therapy

Several institutions with large brachytherapy programs are using HDR units in shielded operating rooms for intraoperative radiation therapy. These programs combine surgery and radiation oncology. The tumor is exposed and a single fraction of radiation is delivered through the open wound. These programs are usually only available in institutions that can commit the resources necessary to build a dedicated brachytherapy operating-room suite. The radiation safety issues in these facilities and shielding design have been discussed in some publications (Anderson et al., 1999; Sephton et al., 1999).

4.9.4   Balloon Applicators

Some techniques rely on balloon applicators for treatment of malignant resection cavity margins. The standard of care for brain tumors, particularly gliomas, has been ERT with or without the additional implantation of ^{125}I seeds. This technique relies on the installation of an organically-based liquid labeled with activities up to 18.5 GBq (500 mCi) of ^{125}I into a balloon previously placed in the surgical cavity at the time the tumor was excised (Dempsey *et al.*, 1998). The organic liquid and the balloon are then withdrawn after several days of treatment. The radiation safety considerations for this treatment are more typical of radiopharmaceutical therapy and include contamination concerns and radioactive waste disposal. Another consideration is the possibility of radioiodinated molecules leaking out of a ruptured balloon or diffusing through the balloon membrane into the cavity and being de-iodinated to liberate radioiodide which is then transported to and concentrated in the thyroid (DeGuzman *et al.*, 2003; Strzelczyk and Safadi, 2004). The use of this technique is currently limited to some larger centers capable of the delicate surgery involved. However, if this technique is successful in significant groups of patients, its use may be expanded to smaller facilities.

5. Facility Design

Radiation sources used in brachytherapy and radiopharmaceutical therapy have the potential to contribute significant doses to medical personnel and others who may spend time within or adjacent to rooms that contain radiation sources or patients administered various types of radiation sources. Meaningful dose reduction can be achieved through the use of appropriate facility design. While the radiation sources used in both brachytherapy and radiopharmaceutical therapy may pose unique radiation safety issues, facilities may be designed to protect against radiation from a variety of sources used in both modalities. This Section will discuss separately the design of facilities used for brachytherapy and radiopharmaceutical therapy, but facilities may be used for both purposes when their design satisfies the safety considerations for both types of therapy. This Section provides recommendations on facility design that may be useful in reducing potential radiation exposure from sources that are being prepared, are in storage, or are being administered to or are within hospitalized patients.

5.1 General Considerations

Section 1 of NCRP Report No. 147 (NCRP, 2004a) and Section 1 of NCRP Report No. 151 (NCRP, 2005) discuss quantities and units, shielding design goals, and effective dose. While neither of these reports directly addresses the subject of shielding design for brachytherapy facilities, the basic principles discussed in Section 1 of both reports will apply to brachytherapy and radiopharmaceutical therapy. The shielding design recommendations in these reports reflect the principles outlined in NCRP Report No. 116 (NCRP, 1993b).

A "controlled area" is a limited-access area in which the occupational exposure of personnel to radiation or radioactive material is under the supervision of an individual in charge of radiation protection. This designation implies that access, occupancy and working conditions are controlled for radiation protection purposes. In brachytherapy facilities, such areas are usually in the immediate areas where radiation-producing equipment or sealed sources are used, such as treatment rooms and control consoles, or other areas that require control of access, occupancy and working conditions for radiation protection purposes. The workers in these areas are those individuals who are specifically trained in the use of ionizing radiation and whose radiation exposure is usually individually monitored. "Uncontrolled areas" for radiation protection purposes include all other areas in the hospital or facility and the surrounding environs. Trained radiation-oncology personnel, other trained staff, as well as members of the public, frequent many areas near controlled areas such as examination rooms or restrooms. These areas *should* be treated as uncontrolled for purposes of shielding design.

There are different shielding design goals for controlled and uncontrolled areas. Shielding design goals are practical values for a single brachytherapy or nuclear-medicine source or sets of sources that are evaluated at reference points beyond a protective barrier. The shielding design goals ensure that the respective annual values for effective dose recommended in NCRP Report No. 147 and Report No. 151 (2004a; 2005) for controlled and uncontrolled areas are not exceeded. Shielding design goals are expressed most often as weekly values because the workload for treatment facilities and the length of stay for radiopharmaceutical therapy has traditionally utilized a weekly format.

5.1.1 *Controlled Areas*

NCRP recommends an annual effective dose limit for occupational personnel of 50 mSv y^{-1} with the cumulative effective dose limit not to exceed the product of 10 mSv and the worker's age in years (exclusive of medical exposure received as part of the worker's health care and natural background radiation) (NCRP, 1993b). NCRP also recommends that new and modified medical-radiation facilities *should* be designed to control annual occupational doses to individuals (*i.e.*, in controlled areas) to a fraction of the 10 mSv y^{-1} value implied by the cumulative effective dose limit as discussed in NCRP Report No. 116 (NCRP, 1993b) and Report No. 147 (NCRP, 2004a). Another design consideration is that a pregnant radiation worker *should not* be exposed to levels that result in greater than the monthly equivalent-dose limit of 0.5 mSv to the worker's embryo or fetus (NCRP, 1993b). To achieve these recommendations, NCRP Report No. 147 and No. 151 (NCRP, 2004a; 2005) recommend an annual effective dose value of 5 mSv y^{-1} (one-half of the 10 mSv y^{-1} value), and a weekly shielding design goal of 0.1 mSv dose equivalent (an annual value of 5 mSv dose equivalent). For controlled areas this shielding design goal would allow pregnant radiation workers continued access to their work areas.

Recommendation for Controlled Areas:
Shielding design goal (in dose equivalent):
0.1 mSv week (equivalent to 5 mSv y⁻¹).

5.1.2 *Uncontrolled Areas*

Uncontrolled areas are occupied by individuals such as patients, visitors to the facility (*e.g.*, delivery service, representatives, and consultants) and employees who do not work routinely with or around radiation sources. Areas adjacent to, but not part of the brachytherapy or nuclear-medicine facility may also be designated as uncontrolled areas. Based on recommendations in NCRP Report No. 116 (NCRP, 1993b), recommendations for the annual limit of effective dose to a member of the public, shielding designs *shall* limit exposure of all individuals in uncontrolled areas to an effective dose that does not exceed 1 mSv y⁻¹. The design and use of new or modified medical-radiation facilities *should* be adequate to control the effective dose to members of the public (*i.e.*, in uncontrolled areas) to 1 mSv y⁻¹ (NCRP, 2004a; 2004b). This recommendation can be achieved with a weekly shielding design goal of 0.02 mSv dose equivalent (an annual value of 1 mSv dose equivalent).

Recommendation for Uncontrolled Areas:
Shielding design goal (in dose equivalent):
0.02 mSv week (equivalent to 1 mSv y⁻¹).

A qualified expert *should* participate in the planning, design and acceptance testing of new or modified brachytherapy and radiopharmaceutical-therapy facilities to ensure that appropriate consideration is given to site selection, facility layout, shielding, ventilation, space for preparation and storage of radiation sources, and physical safeguards. Competent review during design and construction will ensure that the facility design will be adequate to permit operation within established safety standards and maintain radiation exposure at levels that are ALARA.

5.1.3 *Designation of Occupational Radiation Employees*

The vast majority of patients who receive temporary implant therapy and some patients who receive permanent implants or radiopharmaceutical therapy need to be confined to a controlled area of the hospital that is staffed by appropriately trained caregivers. These personnel *should* be considered radiation workers if:

- they work directly with radiation sources; or
- they have a reasonable possibility of receiving an annual effective dose exceeding 1 mSv; or
- the potential for a patient incident is non-negligible and failure to bring such an incident under control could result in effective doses >1 mSv to some individual.

In assessing the applicability of these criteria, both the frequency of procedures in question and the intensity of medical care required (basically, the occupancy factor for the nursing staff) *should* be considered. In general, it is not always necessary to room patients in a controlled area when they contain permanent implants of low-energy photon sources such as ^{103}Pd or ^{125}I; beta-emitting radiopharmaceuticals, such as ^{32}P; or smaller amounts of gamma-emitting radiopharmaceuticals for the treatment of benign conditions, such as the use of ^{131}I for treatment of hyperthyroidism. Some patients with temporary implants that contain high activity low-energy sources (*e.g.*, episcleral plaque therapy for intra-ocular malignancies) may not need to be confined to a controlled area. The criteria above may not be met when significant numbers of patients are treated with interstitial and intracavitary implants using ^{137}Cs, ^{192}Ir, high specific activity ^{125}I, or very large doses of gamma-emitting radiopharmaceuticals. However, the situation for each patient *shall* be evaluated by measurement as described in Section 5.1.4.

5.1.4 *Consideration for Patient Areas*

Placing brachytherapy patients or radiopharmaceutical therapy patients in existing, unshielded hospital rooms may expose persons in adjacent areas to an effective dose that >1 mSv during the treatment period. There may also be regulatory requirements for limiting the dose in unrestricted areas that need be met. Several actions can be taken to minimize radiation exposure to persons in adjacent areas, such as evacuation of adjacent patient rooms and use of portable shielding. Radiation measurements *shall* be made after each intervention to confirm that the potential dose is within regulatory limits. Worst case scenarios may be documented and used to demonstrate the conditions under which these limits are satisfied to avoid the necessity of measuring exposure rates in adjacent areas (especially adjacent, occupied patient rooms) during every treatment. The RSO *shall* be consulted to determine whether adjacent rooms *should* be vacated or whether use of portable shielding or other actions could reduce radiation exposures in adjacent areas to acceptable levels.

If the hospital has designated certain rooms for brachytherapy patients, it may be advantageous to use the same rooms for radioiodine inpatients, particularly if these rooms have been shielded. Medical personnel for these rooms *shall* be trained in radiation safety procedures and *shall* be familiar with limitations associated with visitors and ancillary personnel. Facilities that treat a large number of patients may wish to consider installation of structural shielding in designated room(s). The ideal time to install shielding is during new construction. However, shielding can be added at any time to existing rooms in facilities that are capable of supporting the additional weight. Permanent shielding may consist of poured concrete, core filled concrete block, steel plate, or lead sheet. A detailed discussion of the advantages and disadvantages of shielding materials in common use can be found in Section 4.3 of NCRP Report No. 151 (NCRP, 2005). Table B.3 of this Report lists the properties of various shielding materials in common use. Section 4 of this Report also provides shielding details for joints and junctions between barriers and shielding details for duct penetrations that will apply to all facilities. Care *shall* be taken to ensure that voids are adequately shielded.

5.2 Brachytherapy Treatment

Radiation-oncology personnel may be exposed to a variety of radiation sources. Radionuclide sources used in brachytherapy are the most significant source of occupational radiation exposure to radiation-oncology personnel. Occupational and public exposure may occur during receipt, transport and preparation of sources, loading and unloading sources in brachytherapy applicators, and care of patients during the course of treatment.

A brachytherapy facility consists of all dedicated and shared physical and technological resources that are required to plan and deliver sealed-source brachytherapy treatments. A brachytherapy facility may include:

- a treatment planning area;
- an operating room or procedure room in which applicators or sources can be placed in the patient;
- a radiographic imaging system for documenting the location and geometry of the sources and the applicator or catheters;
- a treatment room; and
- a source preparation and storage area for use with LDR implants.

Facilities for treatment of brachytherapy patients fall into two very different groups: conventional LDR inpatient-based therapy and outpatient-based fractionated HDR brachytherapy.

Facility design in both cases is dictated by similar considerations:

- medical and physical well-being of the patient;
- protection of the staff, visitors and other members of the public from actual and potential radiation hazards; and
- geographic and functional integration of treatment delivery with the applicator-insertion, implant-imaging, treatment-planning, and treatment-evaluation activities.

Because of the very large difference in source strength needed for LDR and HDR treatment modalities, the facilities needed, the temporal distribution of treatment, and the magnitude of radiation hazards to be managed are quite different. Each of the various types of brachytherapy is discussed in the following sections.

5.2.1 Treatment-Area Design

Selection criteria and design endpoints for the treatment-delivery area include:

- proximity to specialized nursing and medical inpatient services needed to provide good quality medical care of the patient;
- functional adequacy including floor space needed for shields and any remote afterloading equipment;
- proximity to the operating rooms, imaging facility, and source preparation area;
- proximity to and occupancy of surrounding uncontrolled areas;
- structural integrity of the building needed to support the weight of required structural or portable shielding;
- well-defined areas to house the patient, entry to which by the general public and nonoccupationally-exposed hospital workers can be controlled by the nursing staff. Except for those patients permanently implanted with low-energy photon sources such as ^{103}Pd or ^{125}I, implanted patients *shall* be housed in private rooms. The entire room occupied by an implanted patient *shall* be considered a controlled area.

- protection of members of the public, including nonradioactive patients or nonoccupationally-exposed workers, who frequent the uncontrolled areas surrounding the facility; and

- protection of occupationally-exposed personnel (*e.g.*, nurses, radiation therapists, oncology staff) and other caregivers, who have been designated as radiation workers.

These criteria may be met cost effectively by grouping treatment rooms together in one or two limited areas rather than using individual patient treatment suites throughout the hospital. This approach limits the number of persons who must receive annual training and develops nursing expertise in managing both the safety and clinical aspects of brachytherapy by maximizing procedure frequency. Some hospitals may not wish to admit all implant and radiopharmaceutical therapy patients to a single area of the hospital because such organization may not be consistent with the goal of providing good quality medical care to implanted patients. For example, patients with implants of the oral cavity, tongue and neck may need specialized wound care, and the need to respond quickly to clinical problems may demand nursing skills typically not found in other nursing units. It may be possible to partially address this issue by providing additional training to nurses on a grouped unit or by rotating specially trained nurses through the area that contains the treatment rooms. Individual brachytherapy treatment rooms may be grouped together to the extent that the quality of patient medical care is not compromised. For an institution with a large brachytherapy program where such groupings are not feasible, the development of two or three specialized facilities may be considered in high-volume locations (*e.g.*, gynecologic oncology, otorhinolaryngology, and thoracic surgery).

Implant rooms *should* be selected to minimize both the uncontrolled personnel traffic in and out of the area and the shielding needed to protect surrounding uncontrolled areas. Placing rooms in the corner of a building often avoids the need to shield all walls in the designated room, especially when treatment rooms are not located at street level. Optimally, a dedicated suite of adjacent rooms on both sides of a blind-end corridor can be designated for brachytherapy and the area defined by means of a properly posted door. The entire posted area can be designated as a controlled area. Use of single isolated rooms requires that the hallway and the surrounding adjacent rooms be treated as uncontrolled areas unless they are vacated or occupancy is controlled during the treatment.

The need for structural or portable shielding *shall* be carefully assessed by a qualified expert before placing a brachytherapy or radiopharmaceutical treatment room into service. Appendix D summarizes the considerations for shielding of HDR brachytherapy facilities as well as general considerations in shielding design. Shielding calculations both for controlled and uncontrolled areas *shall* take into account maximal expected workload and occupancy factors. The thickness of a typical hospital floor is from 10 to 15 cm of concrete, a thickness that may limit the workload for certain types of applications (*e.g.*, the use of ^{137}Cs for intracavitary implants). New construction may use sheetrock for interior walls but sheetrock walls provide negligible protection for energetic photon emitters. Older buildings constructed with cinder block or solid concrete block may provide significant radiation shielding. These assessments *should* be made by a qualified expert.

For protection of adjacent rooms, portable lead shields may be used, although it must be recognized that such shields are rarely large enough to confer protection to the entire room. Inpatient beds in adjacent rooms *should* be assigned occupancy factors of 100 % ($T = 1$). Table B.1 of NCRP Report No. 151 (NCRP, 2005) provides suggested occupancy factors for use as a guide in shielding design. The occupancy factor (T) for an area is the average fraction of time that the maximally exposed individual is present. This Report is intended to support shielding design for megavoltage radiations. In these facilities, the treatment beam cycles on and off as patients are treated. However, in brachytherapy and radiopharmaceutical therapy treatment, the source of radiation is continuously present throughout the course of the treatment. Consequently, there will be no application of a "use factor," or fraction of "beam-on" time on a shielded barrier, that can be applied in the design of brachytherapy or radiopharmaceutical therapy facilities.

When using lower occupancy factors, care *should* be taken that the integrated dose within 1 h falls within the applicable regulatory limit for unrestricted areas. Following installation of structural shielding or placement of portable shielding, a radiation survey of the surrounding areas using an appropriately sensitive, calibrated ion-chamber survey meter *shall* be made to confirm the intent of the shielding calculations. If the survey reveals that the shielding is not adequate to satisfy the applicable exposure limits, either the workload or occupancy of the surrounding areas *shall* be limited appropriately. Alternatively the shielding could be augmented if feasible.

Other equipment needed in treatment facilities include portable shields for protection of staff and lead storage containers for use in patient rooms. All rooms occupied by implanted patients or containing supplies of radioactive sources *should* be posted as controlled or restricted areas. Intercom systems *should* be used to reduce the need for entry of patient care and ancillary personnel into the treatment room.

5.2.2 *Low Dose-Rate Conventional Remote Afterloading Systems*

Shielding requirements for uncontrolled areas surrounding the treatment area are unchanged by the use of LDR remote afterloading because the shielding design would be the same as that for nonafterloading systems. The major benefit of LDR remote afterloading is reduction of exposure to nursing and other inpatient personnel who attend the patient. Operationally, the use of LDR remote afterloading avoids the need for portable shielding used solely to protect occupationally-exposed personnel and visitors entering the treatment room. Shielding in the treatment room will not be necessary because anyone entering the treatment room will trigger the source interlocks causing the sources to retract.

Treatment rooms used for LDR remote afterloaded brachytherapy *should* satisfy all relevant requirements for manually afterloaded brachytherapy. In addition:

- additional floor space for positioning the treatment device and any specialized utilities such as dedicated compressed air and power sources may need to be provided;
- door interlock that causes all sources to be retracted whenever the door is opened *shall* be provided. The interlock mechanism *shall not* cause sources to return to treatment positions by closing the door without initiating a treatment resumption command from the control panel. If an operational door interlock system cannot be provided, nursing and medical personnel *shall* be instructed to practice manual afterloading patient procedures, or the room *should* be equipped with an alternative system for verifying source retraction (*e.g.*, an area monitor);
- treatment rooms *shall* be equipped with an independent area monitor that clearly indicates to staff entering the room whether all sources have been retracted upon interrupting treatment; and
- remote afterloaders *shall* be equipped with visual or audible signals that clearly indicate the presence of any error condition that jeopardizes treatment accuracy or staff safety. These signals *shall* be monitored continuously during patient treatment.

5.2.3 *Requirements for Source Preparation and Storage Room*

The source preparation room *shall* include:

- an area where all LDR sealed sources can be safely stored in an orderly fashion;
- space and facilities for receiving and returning sources, calibration of sources, assessment of homogeneity, inventory of sources, and QC tests;
- space and equipment for source preparation for specific patient treatments;
- a work area in or near the preparation room where records can be prepared and stored and not be subject to radioactive contamination;
- space for QA and treatment aids; and
- space, if necessary, for storage of short-lived sources or temporary storage of unused long-lived sources.

The source-preparation room *should* be located near the LDR treatment rooms and *should not* be shared with other functions. The room *shall* be posted with radiation warning signs and equipped with a lock to secure the area from unauthorized entry. A latch *should* automatically lock the door and require a mechanical or electronic key to open the door. A structurally adequate workbench sufficient for supporting the shielding required for personnel and the source safe *should* be in the room. Space for calibration-source homogeneity checks and shielded transport containers *shall* be provided within the source preparation room. Personnel shielding such as a leaded "L-block" *shall* be provided. This shielding *shall* include a leaded window of sufficient thickness that allows the operator to manipulate and visualize LDR brachytherapy sources without significant whole-body or eye exposure. The adequacy of this local shielding system *shall* be verified by a qualified expert before initiating use. Additional space or safes may be needed if unused sources are to be stored. Once the local shielding is in place, an assessment of the protection afforded to surrounding areas *shall* also be performed prior to initiating use. Changes or additions to the local shielding may be necessary based on the results of this assessment. The room *should* be carefully laid out to ensure that occupational doses are maintained ALARA. Local shielding such as interlocking lead blocks to reduce exposure rates during source preparation, record keeping and other work functions *shall* be used throughout the working areas. Occupancy of the area *should* be limited to persons immediately involved in source preparation. The preparation of radioactive sources (*e.g.*, selection and trimming of ^{192}Ir ribbons or loading of intracavitary source inserts) *should* be performed in the source preparation area.

5.2.4 *Low Dose-Rate Procedure Rooms and Treatment-Planning/Imaging Equipment*

Applicator insertion can be performed in any operating room that supports the surgical procedures needed to evaluate the patient's condition and expose the implant site. For many types of procedures, an imaging system (*e.g.*, a radiographic or CT unit) for intraoperative examination of source placement and geometry is highly recommended. This allows implants with suboptimal or poor geometry to be rapidly identified and corrections made while the patient is still in the operating room. Shielding for these systems *should* meet the shielding design goals for medical x-ray imaging facilities specified in NCRP Report No. 147 (NCRP, 2004a).

5.2.5 *Requirements for High Dose-Rate Brachytherapy Facilities*

High dose-rate (HDR) brachytherapy facilities are usually located within the radiation-oncology department and treatments are staffed by radiation-oncology personnel (therapists, dosime-trists and physicists in addition to the radiation oncologist). The size of the facility and accessories needed depend on whether both imaging and applicator insertion will be performed in the treatment room (Glasgow and Corrigan, 1995b). Facilities to be designed range from using space within an existing ERT treatment room in which an HDR unit is placed to an integrated HDR operat-ing room in which applicator insertion, imaging and treatment are executed without moving the patient. Treatment planning may be more complex than that for LDR brachytherapy, ranging from 15 to 30 min for manual calculation for planning of a simple line source, to 1.5 h for complex optimization of an intracavitary insertion, to several hours for a large interstitial implant. Patient treatment loads are typically limited to three to eight HDR procedures per day on a single machine, depending on the complexity of treatment planning required (see Appendix D for a complete discussion of shielding of HDR brachytherapy facilities).

An HDR brachytherapy facility requires a:

- operating or procedure room;
- radiographic imaging system;
- dedicated treatment room; and
- treatment planning area.

The relative proximity of these facilities can significantly influence procedure flow and efficiency. For example, if the treatment planning area is near the HDR control console, the physicist can perform or supervise treatment planning while being available to respond to treatment-machine malfunctions.

There are four major options for a dedicated HDR facility:

- sharing a treatment vault between an HDR remote afterloader and a linear accelerator or teletherapy machine, using existing operating rooms and imaging equipment. If the external-beam equipment is used heavily, the HDR treatment times will be limited and will require careful scheduling among the three resources: treatment room, operating or procedure room, and imaging facility;
- dedicated vault for the HDR unit using existing operating rooms and simulator. A larger patient load, typically from three to five procedures per day, can be sustained. However, the patient must be transported twice (operating or procedure room to simulator and simulator to treatment room), a requirement that reduces efficiency, hinders immobilization of the applicator system, and for some gynecological applicator systems, may result in a higher incidence of organ perforation. Also, a holding area for patients is required;
- dedicated vault in which both applicator insertion and treatment are carried out while imaging is performed elsewhere. If no cervical dilations or other invasive procedures are to be performed, only an appropriate procedure table may be required. However, if regional or general anesthesia is required, along with control of sterility, then a significant investment, including scrub and recovery areas and anesthesia stations, is needed. Other medical staff (*e.g.*, gynecologic oncologist and anesthesiologist) must be committed to supplying medical services outside their usual venue. A significant patient load, from five to eight procedures per day, can be accommodated, depending on the complexity of treatment planning; and
- integrated brachytherapy suite. This option carries the approaches above to their logical conclusion by incorporating a dedicated HDR system into an operating/treatment room. No transport of the patient between applicator insertion and treatment is required affording the ultimate in applicator-system immobilization, treatment-delivery efficiency, patient comfort and protection of the patient from trauma.

The optimal choice among various alternatives depends primarily on the anticipated patient load. The more expensive options *should* be reserved for programs anticipating a load of at least 500 procedures annually or more than three procedures on each day of use. Other considerations are the clinical importance attached to good immobilization and the complexity of treatment planning considered necessary. As an example, if extensive optimization of source positioning and dwell-times is required, the factor limiting patient load may become the time required for treatment planning and dose calculation rather than the design of the facility. Close cooperation among the radiation oncologist, the physicist, and other involved medical personnel is essential to identify the design criteria and to design a facility that meets the medical facility's needs for the least capital investment. No single design serves all needs, because the design process is driven by so many facility-specific logistical and clinical constraints.

The essential safety features of an HDR treatment room are:

- *properly shielded area*: As discussed in Section 5.1, for adjacent uncontrolled areas, shielding *shall* be designed to limit the annual effective dose to members of the public, including nonradioactive patients, to 1 mSv as a result of brachytherapy procedures. For surrounding controlled areas, shielding *shall* be designed to control occupational exposures to the annual dose value specified by an institution's ALARA program. Portable shields *shall not* be used for this purpose. The adequacy of the proposed or existing shielding design *shall* be reviewed by a qualified expert. Before implementing an HDR treatment program or otherwise accumulating significant integrated dose, the dose rates in surrounding areas *shall* be measured using a properly calibrated ion-chamber survey meter [see Section 6 of NCRP Report No. 151 (NCRP, 2005) for a discussion of surveys]. The survey results *shall* be reviewed by a qualified expert. If the results indicate that the applicable effective dose values could be exceeded, the facility *shall* limit the patient treatment workload, augment the shielding, or appropriately limit occupancy in surrounding areas to prevent the applicable values from being exceeded.
- *secure area*: Considerations regarding security of these areas have become an increasing cause of concern following the events of September 11, 2001. The potential for sources used in HDR units to be stolen and placed in so-called "dirty bombs" has caused many facilities to substantially increase

the level of security for these areas. When not supervised by trained personnel, the HDR facility or treatment facility *shall* be secured to prevent inadvertent exposure of individuals and tampering with the HDR unit itself. The security plan including the locks on such a room *shall* be reviewed with a security expert. Keys for the facility *should* be separate from master keys for other areas in the facility and the use of card access, fingerprint scanning, or other security measures *should* be part of the overall security plan. Access to the units, including the provision of keys, *should* be under the immediate control of the physics or radiation-oncology staff and the number of persons present at the units *should* be limited and under the immediate supervision of the radiation-oncology staff. Access to the operator's key for the control console *should* be controlled by the radiation-oncology staff and restricted to a list of specific individuals. In addition to access controls, consideration *should* also be given to fastening down the units themselves to prevent relocation or theft. Plans to implement these measures *should* be reviewed with a security expert.

- *engineered/administrative controls such as*:
  - a door interlock system that causes the source to retract upon opening the door;
  - an independent area monitor visible at the entrance;
  - appropriate radiation warning signs;
  - "beam-on" light that is activated whenever the source is in the exposed position;
  - systems for maintaining visual and aural contact with the patient during treatment (*e.g.*, television monitoring systems and two-way intercom systems);
  - a copy of the operator's manual, including all relevant procedures for operation of the device, written emergency procedures, and explanations of all error codes, placed near the operator's console;
  - fault detection logic capable of detecting source retraction failure, separation of the source from its cable, and unscheduled displacement of the source from its programmed treatment position or position in the shielded safe. Such fault detection logic *should* alert users to the problem and prevent further treatment. Error-detection and recovery systems located on the HDR afterloader *shall* be thoroughly tested before implementing a clinical treatment program and *should* be tested at appropriate intervals thereafter;

- emergency procedures *shall* be developed for quickly detecting HDR source retraction failures and bringing the source under control. These procedures *shall* include use of a radiation survey meter to confirm source containment, use of a cable cutter and tools to safely manipulate the source, and emergency removal of the applicators if needed. Equipment needed to implement these procedures, such as a shielded storage container, forceps, cable cutters, etc., *shall* be present whenever the device is used; and
- a calibrated survey meter, capable of detecting source exposure in the presence of HDRs. The survey meter *shall* be available whenever the HDR remote afterloader is used).

In calculating required shielding, workloads *should* be estimated conservatively (*i.e.*, in the safe direction) and *should* include source exposures anticipated for QA, source calibration, and other measurements. A moderately large workload might be estimated at 100 patients per year with an average between three to five treatment fractions per patient. It is usual to assume that the workload will be evenly distributed throughout the year. Therefore, it is reasonable to design a barrier to meet the weekly shielding design goals discussed in Section 5.1. Treatment rooms are often constructed below ground level as the most economic strategy for reducing shielding costs. For rooms below ground (below grade), the costs of excavation, when necessary, sealing against water and provision for access need to be considered in light of the overall cost.

When HDR units are placed within existing linear accelerator vaults, it can usually be safely assumed that no additional shielding is necessary. However, placing the unit in such a room will mean that for a portion of the treatment week, patients cannot be treated on the linear accelerator. For a dedicated HDR treatment room, 40 to 60 cm of concrete or from 5 to 7 cm of lead would typically be required to adequately shield uncontrolled areas, depending on the location of the source relative to the areas under consideration and the occupancy of the adjacent areas. Every wall, the ceiling, and the floor in the HDR treatment room *shall* serve as a primary barrier. Although primary-beam teletherapy shielding is usually more than adequate, existing teletherapy barriers, including the door to the facility, designed only to protect against scattered and leakage radiation may not be adequate for HDR brachytherapy. If the HDR source location is not fixed to a single location in the room, the influence of source position on shielding efficacy *shall* be evaluated by a qualified expert. If the shielding design restricts the source to a designated location within the room, the location *shall* be permanently marked or otherwise fixed on the floor.

As noted above, following installation of the HDR remote afterloader, the adequacy of all shielding barriers *shall* be confirmed by a qualified expert performing an appropriate facility survey. Sections 6.1, 6.2 and 6.3 of NCRP Report No. 151 (NCRP, 2005) can be applied to HDR facilities. Thereafter, surveys *should* be performed at appropriate intervals or whenever changes in surrounding space utilization, HDR workload, positioning of the remote afterloader, or modifications to the structural shielding call into question the adequacy of the existing survey.

5.2.6 *Additional Requirements for "Pulsed" Dose-Rate Brachytherapy Facilities*

Pulsed dose-rate (PDR) units have been suggested as substitutes for LDR applications. In principle, PDR brachytherapy requires no additional shielding above that required for the corresponding continuous LDR implant, because the average hourly absorbed-dose rate, in Gy m^2 h^{-1}, and total treatment absorbed dose, in Gy m^2, are unchanged. Shielding requirements could decrease if a PDR ^{192}Ir source is used to replace conventional sources of ^{137}Cs. Use of large pulse widths for several days may make it possible to exceed the shielding design goal of 1 mSv y^{-1} for uncontrolled areas. Before implementing a PDR brachytherapy treatment, the user *shall* evaluate the average hourly and weekly exposures to determine that the proposed dwell-time per pulse and cumulative dwell-time will not result in exceeding the appropriate shielding design goals for controlled and uncontrolled areas. Specific procedures for implementing this requirement have been published (Williamson *et al.*, 1995).

5.3 Facilities for Unsealed Sources

Nuclear-medicine personnel receive occupational exposure from numerous radionuclide sources, including those used in therapeutic applications. Commonly used radionuclides in therapeutic nuclear medicine include beta emitters (*e.g.*, ^{90}Y and ^{32}P) and photon sources (*e.g.*, ^{131}I) (Tables 3.1, 3.2, and 3.3). While energetic beta emitters may contribute to significant hand doses during handling, such sources do not contribute significantly to whole-body radiation exposure. On the other hand, energetic, penetrating gamma radiation may contribute significant whole-body doses to personnel. In terms of facility design, beta emitters pose a negligible external exposure hazard. Exposure from photon emitters will need to be reduced by adequate facility design.

5.3.1 Radiopharmaceutical Dispensing Laboratory

It is unlikely that a laboratory will be designed only for therapeutic purposes and the design of the laboratory *shall* consider the diagnostic and therapeutic applications in use in the facility. In general, if the dispensing laboratory or nuclear pharmacy has been designed for the use of radioiodine, in particular ^{131}I, it will generally provide adequate protection for use of other radiopharmaceuticals. However, the overall laboratory design *shall* be reviewed by a qualified expert. A fume hood *shall* be equipped with a charcoal-filtered exhaust to capture any radioiodine that is vaporized during the dispensing procedure. The fume hood *shall* be certified and have an appropriate flow velocity (typically from ~100 to 150 linear ft min^{-1}). Concentration of radioiodine in exhaust gas *shall* be reviewed at least annually to verify that concentrations released to the atmosphere are below any applicable regulatory limits. In addition to the shielding provided by the original shipping container, additional local shielding may be necessary to protect personnel who dispense therapeutic radiopharmaceuticals as well as personnel in adjacent rooms. Exposure-rate measurements *shall* be conducted in adjacent areas to confirm that radiation doses are ALARA (NCRP, 1998). Personnel who work in the dispensing laboratory *shall* use adequate physical safeguards to maintain radiation exposures to themselves and others ALARA. Physical safeguards include all physical devices used to restrict access of staff and other individuals to radiation sources or to reduce radiation levels as described in NCRP Report No. 71 (NCRP, 1983). Such physical safeguards may include: shielding (generally lead), long tongs or forceps for handling radioactive sources, "warning" signage and postings, locks, and audible and visual alarms integrated into radiation monitoring equipment. Protective devices used to minimize uptake of radionuclides include: protective clothing such as laboratory coats, protective eyewear, disposable gloves, sleeve protectors, shoe covers, aprons, plastic-backed absorbent pads, water-tight containers (*e.g.*, spill-proof vials with crimped rubber septa), glove boxes, high exchange-rate room exhaust systems, fume hoods equipped with trapping filters, and respiratory protection devices. Radioactively contaminated disposable or nondisposable items *shall* be treated appropriately and held for decay in storage in a properly designed area or disposed of as radioactive waste.

Security of a radiopharmacy, and the radioactive materials contained in it *shall* be reviewed by a security expert. Access to the radiopharmacy *should* be restricted to nuclear-medicine staff dispensing the radiopharmaceuticals. Delivery of stock materials from a radiopharmacy off-site *should* require that the materials received be placed in a locked, secure area until the radiopharmacy staff moves the materials to their final destinations. Coded access to these areas and other procedures to limit access *shall* be in place. Receipt of shipments off-hours may require specific training for receiving or security personnel by the facility radiation safety staff.

5.3.2 *Storage of Low-Level Radioactive Waste*

The types of wastes generated by the therapeutic applications of radioactive materials will generally fall into four categories:

- sealed sources whose activities have decayed below the levels required for clinical use;
- materials contaminated during preparation of therapeutic radiopharmaceuticals;
- patient wastes (excluding patient excreta); and
- medical wastes containing small amounts of radioactive materials.

Sealed sources will not present problems of contamination, but will require storage for long periods (*i.e.*, periods up to or exceeding 2 y) depending on their half-lives. The amount of storage space needed will vary depending on the size of the overall program including unsealed sources. The sources may need to be stored in shielded containers to reduce the exposure rates in adjacent areas. A general discussion of management techniques for low-level radioactive waste is beyond the scope of this Report, but this topic is discussed in NCRP Report No. 143 (NCRP, 2003). Volume reduction of low-level radioactive wastes *should* be practiced whenever possible. Such reduction is not only based on economics and ALARA principles but on the necessity of good stewardship of the limited resources available.

Patient wastes generated from radiopharmaceutical therapies may need to be stored for decay for periods from one week to several months depending on the activity used and the identity of the radionuclides used. Provision for the storage of patient wastes *should* include consideration of the overall volumes involved and the possibility of structural shielding being necessary. Designers of a waste handling area may also need to consider the infection control issues associated with contaminated medical wastes including syringes, needles, intravenous tubing, and blood. Such wastes may require engineered spaces and refrigeration in certain situations.

Institutions with large radiopharmaceutical therapy programs can accumulate substantial volumes of contaminated linen and waste that when grouped in one location may represent a large diffuse source of radiation. Centralized waste depots may require the use of portable or structural shielding which *should* be specified by a qualified expert. To minimize the storage of some spent sealed sources (*e.g.*, ^{125}I seeds or ^{192}Ir seeds in ribbons), it may be possible to return these sources to the vendor. When not feasible, localized portable shielding such as lead bricks may provide sufficient shielding. However, because these sources may have relatively long half-lives such storage may be necessary for several years. Sources *should* be stored until the radionuclides have decayed by 10 half-lives or until a survey conducted by radiation safety staff indicates that only background levels of activity are present.

6. Changes in Medical Status of the Radioactive Patient

The decision to treat a patient with brachytherapy or radiopharmaceutical therapy *shall* involve consideration of the ability of the patient to comply with radiation precautions and the patient's overall medical condition. In the event of deterioration in the patient's medical condition, frequent or continual monitoring of the patient may be necessary. Examples of such cases include septic shock, pulmonary edema, and myocardial infarction. If a patient's condition deteriorates significantly, the patient may need to be transferred to intensive, special care, or cardiac care units where special monitoring is available. Typically, patients in these units are in close proximity to each other with little or no shielding available, and may present a radiation hazard to other patients or to patient-care personnel. The radiation oncologist or nuclear-medicine physician and the RSO *shall* be notified of the transfer to a special unit as soon as possible, preferably before the transfer takes place. If a patient is being treated with a temporary implant, the radiation oncologist *should* consider whether the sources *should* be removed. The RSO or designee *shall* determine whether portable shielding is needed to reduce doses to other patients or to patient-care personnel and whether personal monitoring is necessary. The RSO or designee *shall* provide information on radiation precautions necessary to keep radiation exposures to patient-care personnel ALARA.

6.1 Cardiac or Respiratory Arrest

Lifesaving efforts *shall* take precedence over consideration of radiation exposures received by medical personnel. The medical emergency *shall* be declared as soon as the life-threatening event is discovered, and lifesaving efforts *shall* begin immediately. Personnel in the room *should* be limited to those persons necessary for medical management. The RSO *shall* be notified as soon as is feasible. If the patient is being treated with a temporary implant, the radiation oncologist *should* be notified immediately to determine whether the sources should be removed. Patients treated with permanent seed implants generally do not present a radiation hazard to medical personnel responding to a code.

In the case of a patient treated with a therapeutic amount of a liquid radiopharmaceutical <48 h prior to an emergency, it *should* be assumed that body fluid samples contain activity. The dilution of the concentration of activity by the volume of circulating blood will usually be large enough so that the activity in any single sample is below exempt amounts (*i.e.*, amounts of radioactive material so low that the NRC exempts them from regulatory control). Life-saving efforts may result in contamination of the hands or gloves and clothing of medical personnel performing this procedure. These personnel *should not* be allowed to leave the area of the medical emergency until radiation safety personnel have decontaminated the persons involved. Decontamination of the location where the medical emergency has taken place may also be necessary, and *should* be undertaken by radiation safety staff once the medical emergency has been resolved.

6.2 Mental Status of the Patient

Evaluation of the ability of a patient to follow radiation safety instructions *shall* be an integral element in the overall treatment plan. If the patient is disoriented, uncooperative or violent, the patient may attempt to remove the sources or applicator or attempt to leave the facility. The attending physician *should* consider whether sedation or restraint is justified in such cases. The cooperation of patient-care personnel is essential, and all persons caring for the patient *should* be involved in discussion of the treatment plan. Patients with a history of substance abuse may, under the stress of treatment, experience a psychotic episode. These patients *should* be monitored carefully to anticipate any problems.

6.3 Emergency Surgery

If a patient containing therapeutic amounts of radionuclides requires emergency surgery, consideration of radiation exposure *should not* deter the surgery from proceeding. Preparation for the surgery *should* include consultation with the attending radiation oncologist or nuclear-medicine physician and the RSO. If this is not possible and the situation is life-threatening, the surgery *should* proceed and necessary information *should* be conveyed to the surgical team as soon as the attending radiation oncologist or nuclear-medicine physician and the RSO are available. It is not likely that an individual surgeon will perform an appreciable number of procedures on patients who contain therapeutic quantities of radio-active materials. The RSO *should* consider whether or not to issue personal monitors to operating room staff. It is unlikely that doses to operating room personnel from emergency surgeries will approach the annual recommended limit of 5 mSv for infrequent radiation exposures to individual members of the public. However, rotation of operating room personnel *should* be considered in cases where the individual effective dose is likely to exceed 1 mSv from any single procedure. The number of persons in the operating room *should* be minimized, and operating room personnel *should* only remain in the operating room for the minimum amount of time consistent with the surgical objectives.

In the case of treatment with radiopharmaceuticals, if it is estimated that the circulating blood or the area of the body to be treated surgically contains a significant quantity of the radiopharmaceutical, the RSO and the surgeon *should* discuss the procedures to be performed to keep radiation exposure to surgical personnel ALARA. Standard precautions always used in surgical settings will minimize the spread of radioactive contamination and the risk of internal contamination to operating room personnel. Any surgical specimens sent for pathological examination *should* be monitored for contamination. Tools and other equipment from the surgery *should* be monitored for radioactive contamination, decontaminated as necessary, and stored for radioactive decay or treated as radioactive waste. If an injury such as a cut or puncture occurs or a glove is torn during surgery, radioactive contamination of the skin or wound may occur. In addition to the ordinary treatment and follow-up as with any wound, the RSO *shall* be consulted to evaluate any possible radiation hazard, especially internal intake.

6.4 Patients on Dialysis

The administration of therapeutic doses of radiopharmaceuticals to patients on dialysis raises special issues. These patients will not clear radioactive materials as quickly as other patients, and the clearance will generally not take place until the patient undergoes a dialysis session. The decision as to the activity required for such patients *should* be based on a trial administration of activity. Based on the observed elimination rate, the appropriate total activity can be administered to provide the radiation dose required for the treatment. The largest amount of activity will usually be eliminated during the first dialysis session with decreasing amounts eliminated during subsequent sessions. The RSO *should* assess the radiation exposures likely to be received by persons caring for the patient during the dialysis sessions and issue personal monitors as judged necessary. The materials, tubing, filters and waste containers, used during the dialysis session *should* be checked by the RSO to see if these materials need to be removed as low-level radioactive waste. The tubing, filters and waste containers *should* be stored for decay and then disposed in an appropriate manner. The volume of fluids used during these sessions *should* be sufficient to dilute the radioactive concentrations to amounts below regulatory limits for sewer discharge. Thus, these liquid wastes are being treated in the same manner as patient excreta.

6.5 Transfer to Another Healthcare Facility

Subsequent to treatment, patients may be transferred to another healthcare facility (*i.e.*, another hospital, skilled nursing facility, nursing home, or hospice). These patients would most likely contain residual ^{131}I from treatment of benign or malignant thyroid disease or ^{125}I/^{103}Pd permanent interstitial seed implants. Patients being transferred to another healthcare facility *shall* meet the criteria for unrestricted release. The facility accepting the transfer would not need a license for radioactive materials to accept the patient although some facilities may possess such a license. In the case of patients treated with radiopharmaceutical therapy, the possibility for the generation of low-level radioactive waste *should* be examined by the RSO of the treating facility and any issues *should* be discussed with the facility accepting the patient transfer. In the rare event that a patient being transferred to another healthcare facility does not meet the criteria for unrestricted release, the RSO *shall* ensure that the admitting facility has an appropriate license that will allow acceptance of the patient. Many facilities have adopted the policy of issuing a wallet identification card or other means of identification to patients who are released while still containing measurable amounts of radioactive material. Information on such identification documents *should* include the radionuclide used and a telephone number at the treating facility that can be contacted on a 24 h basis, as necessary. The healthcare institution receiving the patient may ask the treating physician or the RSO of the treating institution to provide radiation safety information and precautions, if any, for the patient and for the receiving healthcare facility, including exposures to be expected for personnel who care for the patient. Information provided in such cases *should* include precautions for minimizing external radiation exposure. In the event of radiopharmaceutical administrations, most likely the use of ^{131}I therapies, advice on the use of standard precautions to minimize risk of internal contamination *should* be given by the nuclear-medicine physician or the RSO.

6.6 Readmission of Patients to the Treating Institution

When a patient who still contains a therapeutic quantity of radioactive material is readmitted to the treating hospital, the RSO *shall* be notified as soon as possible after admission. In institutions treating significant numbers of patients, consideration *should* be given to the addition of information on dates of cessation of radiation precautions in electronic chart systems which could be useful in the event of readmission. The RSO *shall* monitor the patient and specify the precautions, if any, to be followed by patient-care personnel. A new complete set of radiation precaution tags *should* be placed on the patient, the patient's room, and chart at the time of this monitoring.

6.7 Death of the Patient

Therapeutic amounts of radioactive materials are not usually administered to moribund patients, although there may be circumstances where the palliative use of radioactive materials in terminal patients will significantly improve the quality-of-life of the patient. The treating physician needs to weigh these quality-of-life issues in making treatment decisions.

6.7.1 *Death of the Patient Within a Treating Facility*

In the rare event that a patient dies in the treating facility while still containing a therapeutic quantity of radioactive material, the treating radiation oncologist or nuclear-medicine physician and the RSO *shall* be notified immediately. In the case of therapeutic radiopharmaceuticals, if several days have elapsed between radiopharmaceutical treatment and death, the radiation hazard may be reduced considerably, and precautions, if any, for handling the body may be minimal.

6.7.2 *Removal of Temporary Implants*

If the body contains a temporary implant, the radiation oncologist *shall* remove the sources prior to transfer of the body to the morgue or funeral home. After the sources have been removed, the RSO or designee *shall* perform a radiation survey to confirm that no sources remain in the body or the hospital room. When it is confirmed that all sources have been retrieved, postmortem care can be initiated.

6.7.3 *Death of the Patient Outside of the Treating Facility*

In most cases, if a patient who has been treated with therapeutic quantities of radioactive materials dies outside the treating medical facility, no special precautions are generally necessary for embalming or other preparation of the body for burial. Patients treated with seed implants will not usually represent a radiation hazard to persons dealing with the body unless there is to be an autopsy or cremation (see Section 6.7.6 for precautions during autopsy and Section 6.7.10 for a discussion of cremation of bodies containing permanent implants). External exposure rates will be minimal, and there is no radioactive contamination. For therapeutic radiopharmaceutical administrations, radioactive contamination from body fluids will be minimal using standard aspiration and injection methods for embalming. The treating physician *should* instruct families of patients who receive >1 GBq of ^{131}I that if the patient expires within 2 d after receiving the treatment, the pathologist or funeral-home personnel receiving the body *should* seek advice from the treating physician or the RSO on methods to keep their radiation exposures ALARA.

6.7.4 *Organ Donation*

If organ donation is a consideration, the RSO *shall* determine necessary precautions for surgical personnel who will harvest the organ(s). It is highly unlikely that the donated organ will contain a quantity of radioactive material sufficient to cause significant damage to the organ or deliver a radiation dose to the recipient sufficient to nullify the donation. The radiation oncologist, nuclear-medicine physician, or RSO *should* be prepared to provide estimates of radiation doses that may be received by the recipient as a result of the transplant. Because the organ donation may be a life-saving event for the organ recipient or may significantly improve the recipient's quality-of-life, a limit for effective dose to the recipient is not required. Any temporary implants *shall* be removed from the body as expeditiously as possible to facilitate organ harvesting. If a delay in removal of the temporary implants is unavoidable, the RSO *shall* determine any interventions, such as portable shielding, necessary to maintain personnel radiation exposures ALARA.

6.7.5 *Permanent Implants and Radiopharmaceuticals*

If the patient was treated with a permanent implant or with a therapeutic amount of a radiopharmaceutical, the "radiation precaution" wristband *should* remain on the body and an additional tag *should* be placed on the outside of the shroud. If several days have elapsed between the radiopharmaceutical treatment and death, the radiation hazard will usually be reduced considerably, and radiation safety precautions, if any, may be minimal. The radioactive half-lives of radionuclides used in permanent implants is usually sufficiently long such that the activity will not be reduced significantly. In any event, the RSO *shall* notify the morgue prior to the arrival of the body, and the RSO *should* discuss radiation safety precautions with morgue personnel prior to postmortem procedures.

6.7.6 *Precautions During Autopsy*

As long as the body remains unopened, any radiation exposure received by personnel near the body will be due to gamma rays that penetrate the body from the therapeutic radiation sources. In some cases, the patient may have had a nuclear-medicine procedure prior to death (*e.g.*, a scan for pulmonary embolus) which may contribute to the gamma dose rate. Nuclear-medicine records *should* be checked by the RSO if this is suspected. Patients treated with seed implants will have the radioactive source localized to the area where the seeds were implanted. The RSO or radiation oncologist can advise the pathologist where the seeds are located and that area can be excised before the rest of the autopsy proceeds. Migration of seeds initially implanted in the prostate has been reported in the literature (Merrick *et al.*, 2000; Nag *et al.*, 1997). The pathologist *should* be made aware of this possibility so that seeds found outside the prostate can be excised if possible. The excised tissue can be placed on a separate table. Sectioning of the excised tissue can be done immediately with radiation safety assistance so that any seeds can be removed from sections saved for pathological examination. The excised area including the seeds can then be replaced in the body at the conclusion of the autopsy. It *should* be emphasized to pathology personnel that there is no contamination of body fluids with seed implants. However, it is possible to slice through seeds during sectioning of an excised tissue. The pathologist *should* be warned of this possibility and advised to proceed cautiously.

It is rare that the body of a patient will be delivered to autopsy shortly after administration of a therapeutic radiopharmaceutical. If death occurred shortly after administration (*i.e.*, within 24 to 48 h) a considerable amount of activity will be present in blood and urine. In such cases, the autopsy *should* be supervised by the RSO or designee and personal monitors may be issued to pathology personnel according to the judgment of the RSO. Tissue samples taken by the pathologist for analysis *should* be held until the activity has decayed below measurable levels (*e.g.*, for 10 half-lives). Determination of any residual activity in tissue samples *should* be made by the RSO before release of the samples to the laboratory. If death occurred at any time >48 h post-administration, it can be expected that there will be little, if any, activity in blood or urine, and that the activity will be present only in residual thyroid tissue, if any, or in metastatic disease sites. Personal monitors may be issued to pathology personnel according to the judgment of the RSO. Tissue samples *should* be handled as described above.

In cases where the patient had received a dose of a beta-emitting colloid (*e.g.*, ^{32}P chromic phosphate into a body cavity) activity will have been deposited on serous surfaces with considerable activity remaining in the cavity fluid. During autopsy as much fluid as possible *should* be removed from body cavities before and immediately after the body is opened. The fluid may be washed down the drain in accordance with the instructions of the RSO. Adequate protection against contamination is provided by following precautions necessary for infection control (*e.g.*, protective clothing, gloves, etc.). Any beta radiation emitted by the source will be largely absorbed in superficial tissues. Once the body cavity is opened, however, the beta radiation can expose the pathologist and others who assist in the autopsy. While beta radiation will not penetrate more than a few millimeters into the skin, the dose to hands may be significant because they will be in close contact with body tissues and fluids (Laughlin, 1968). Autopsy personnel *should* wear double gloves to reduce the hand dose from beta emitters. Safety goggles *should* be worn to prevent an accidental splash into the eyes. Goggles typically worn for the purpose of protecting against blood-borne pathogen exposure are usually satisfactory. Specimens from patients treated with radiopharmaceuticals may have to be stored for decay before release for pathological examination. The release of such specimens *should* be under the control of the RSO.

6.7.7 *Preparation for Burial Without Autopsy or Embalming*

If the attending radiation oncologist, nuclear-medicine physician, or RSO believes that the effective dose likely to be received by personnel preparing the body for burial without autopsy or embalming will approach 5 mSv, the treating physicians or RSO *should* provide radiation precaution information to the family of the deceased. In most cases, precautions will be limited to restricting the time spent near the body to provide reasonable assurance that family members will not receive >5 mSv effective dose.

6.7.8 *Preparation for Burial by Embalming*

The administering physician or RSO *should* notify the morgue or funeral home that the body contains therapeutic quantities of radioactive material and *should* provide personnel who embalm the body with precautions to minimize radiation exposure and radioactive contamination. If the maximal dose-equivalent rate at 30 cm from any surface of the body is <0.5 mSv h^{-1}, no special precautions are necessary. Embalming is conducted by injecting an embalming fluid into the body and flushing body fluids into the drain. During the embalming of bodies that contain therapeutic radiopharmaceuticals, personnel involved in the procedure *should* follow precautions similar to those used for infection control (*i.e.*, use of gloves and protective clothing) to avoid personal contamination. Careful cleaning of equipment in the usual manner will remove radioactive contamination. When embalming bodies that contain permanent implants such as ^{125}I or ^{103}Pd, personnel *should* avoid standing next to the area of the body that contains the implant. The RSO *should* discuss the exposure rates to personnel involved in the embalming procedure and provide guidance on the times and distances. It is recommended that the effective dose to personnel be limited to 0.25 mSv per embalmed body.

6.7.9 *Precautions During Visitation*

In most cases, no precautions will be necessary during visitation. If the possibility exists of measurable exposure rates at a distance of 30 cm from the body, the family *should* be given appropriate advice that will provide reasonable assurance that family members will not receive >5 mSv.

6.7.10 *Cremation*

Recommendations in this Section assume that the body has been prepared in accordance with recommendations in the preceding sections. No additional handling precautions are necessary in transporting the body to the crematorium. In cases where the radionuclide-therapy patient dies outside the treating facility, families *should* inform crematorium personnel that the body might contain activity. Crematorium personnel *should* contact the radiation oncologist, nuclear-medicine physician, or RSO if they want additional guidance on handling the body. The physician may refer the questions to the RSO who *should* also provide assistance in decontamination of the crematorium, if necessary.

In cases where the patient dies in a hospital and still contains significant quantities of radiopharmaceuticals, the RSO *should* advise crematorium personnel that the body is radioactive and *should* provide guidance on methods to minimize radiation exposure, contamination of the retort, and especially methods to minimize radioactive ash particles. Modern crematories use a combination of high temperature and forced air to ensure complete combustion of all soft tissues. The only residue consists of finely divided bone ash. Therefore, several types of hazards *should* be considered. The most likely hazard to the general population in the vicinity of the crematorium is the inhalation of radioactive material emitted with the stack gases. Crematorium employees may receive external exposure from the radioactive body or from contamination of the crematorium or internal exposure from inhalation of radioactive particles while handling the ashes (Que, 2001; Wallace, 1991).

The most likely exposure to members of the public would be from cremation of a body that contained ^{131}I. If a crematorium were to handle bodies that contain a total quantity not exceeding 100 GBq in a single year, the effective dose to individuals in the surrounding population would not be likely to exceed 0.1 mSv. While the embalmed body of a radioiodine patient could contain as much as several gigabecquerel of ^{131}I, it is most likely that bodies would contain significantly <0.1 GBq. Therefore, it appears that no radiation hazard would exist even if a crematorium were to handle several bodies per year containing ^{131}I. Approximately 200,000 patients receive ^{131}I therapy per year across the United States (Hundahl, 1998). It is rare for a patient to die during treatment, and it is highly unlikely that a single crematorium would handle >10 bodies that contain therapeutic quantities of ^{131}I.

Bodies that contain gamma-emitting radionuclides will result in some external exposure to employees of the crematorium. Because minimal time is required to handle the body at the crematorium, no precautions are necessary to protect from external radiation exposure. Cremation of bodies that contain radionuclides that are not volatile may result in contamination of the retort. The most significant hazard from this contamination is inhalation of ash particles during cleaning of the retort. The presence of radioactive seeds within a body scheduled to be cremated raises the issue of whether such seeds will be intermixed with ashes upon completion of the process. Because of the very high temperatures used in modern crematoria, it is most probable that the seeds themselves will burst releasing any contained activity into the plume.

Some states and municipalities have proposed restrictions on the number of bodies containing radioactive seeds to be accepted for cremation at any one location or have proposed that the family seek specific permission for cremation of such a body before the cremation can actually take place (Que, 2001). If there are concerns on the part of the family of the deceased about the potential for residual activity in the ashes of the deceased, the RSO of the treating facility *should* be available for consultation and monitoring as deemed necessary. Cremation of bodies that contained beta-emitting radionuclides would be expected to create similar hazards. To prevent significant inhalation of ash particles, workers who clean the retort *should* wear dust masks and protective garments during handling of the ashes and cleaning of the retort. It is unlikely that any crematorium would in any 1 y handle a sufficient number of radioactive bodies such that the radiation doses to workers or the public would exceed 1 mSv. However, each crematorium *should* maintain records of the type and activity in bodies cremated, when known.

Appendix A

Patient-Release Criteria

Sections 3 and 4 of this Report contain patient-release criteria in general terms. This Appendix is intended to present the analytical basis for calculating the pertinent exposure rates and related dose quantities for implementing patient-release criteria applicable to radiopharmaceutical therapy. Although the principles in this Appendix can be applied to brachytherapy, this discussion deals only with radiopharmaceutical therapy. Appendix B presents three specific examples of the application of these principles.

A.1 Dosimetry

Two types of quantities are specifically defined for use in radiological protection: protection quantities, which are defined by ICRP, and operational quantities, which are defined by ICRU. The most recent set of protection quantities recommended in ICRP Publication 60 (ICRP, 1991) includes the effective dose (E) and the tissue or organ equivalent doses (H_T). These quantities are not directly measurable but are amenable to calculation if the conditions of irradiation are known.

Both the protection and operational quantities can be related to the basic physical quantities exposure (X), air kerma (K_a), and tissue absorbed dose (D) (NCRP, 1985). The physical quantities and operational quantities are the basis for measuring external radiation. Exposure (X) is defined as the quotient of dQ by dm, where dQ is the absolute value of the total charge of the ions of one sign produced in air when all the electrons liberated by photons in air having mass dm are completely stopped in air. Air kerma (K_a) is defined as the quotient of dE_{tr} by dm, where dE_{tr} is the sum of the initial kinetic energies of all the charged ionizing particles liberated by uncharged ionizing particles in air having mass dm. The absorbed dose (*D*) is the quotient of dē by d*m*, where dē is the mean energy imparted by ionizing radiation to matter of mass d*m*. The physical quantities and operational quantities are the basis for measuring external radiation.

Conversion coefficients, which relate operational and protection quantities to physical quantities, are calculated using radiation transport codes and the appropriate mathematical models.

A.1.1 *Physical Quantities*

Measurements of the amount of photon radiation emitted from patients are generally made with instruments that are calibrated to indicate exposure (*X*) in roentgens (R). Instruments can also be calibrated in air kerma (K_a) (ICRU, 1998a). Such measurements are made at a point in a radiation field at some specified distance from a patient or shielded enclosure.

The relationship between the quantities air kerma and exposure for photons emitted from treated patients at energies applicable to this Report (0.05 to 1 MeV) is as follows (NIST, 2001):

$$K_a = 0.00876\ X, \tag{A.1}$$

where K_a is expressed in gray and *X* in roentgens. Alternatively, K_a can be obtained by dividing *X* by 114.

For purposes of complying with appropriate shielding design criteria for photons K_a is the recommended quantity (NCRP, 2004b). The absorbed dose (gray) to tissue located at that point is obtained by multiplying the air kerma by 1.099, the mean tissue-to-air mass-energy-absorption coefficient ratio for the applicable photon-energy range (ICRU, 1993).

A.1.2 *Operational Quantities*

The absorbed dose (*D*) at the point of measurement can be modified to account for biological effectiveness of the various radiation types and energies, yielding the operational quantity dose equivalent (*H*) (sieverts) (ICRU, 1993). The dose equivalent (*H*) is product of *D*, *Q* and *N* at the point of interest where *D* is the absorbed dose, *Q* is the quality factor (assigned a value of one for photons), and *N* is the product of all other modifying factors. For individual monitoring the quantity personal dose equivalent [$H_p(d)$] is the dose equivalent in soft tissue, at an appropriate depth (*d*) below a specified point on the body (ICRU, 1993).

A.1.3 *Protection Quantities*

Protection quantities were recommended and defined in ICRP Publication 60 (ICRP, 1991) as well as in NCRP Report No. 82 (NCRP, 1985). These quantities include the organ absorbed dose (D), organ equivalent dose (H_T), and effective dose (E). The effective dose, E, is defined as the sum of the weighted equivalent doses to specific organs or tissues, H_T [*i.e.*, each equivalent dose is weighted by the corresponding tissue weighting factor for the organ or tissue (w_T) (NCRP, 1993)]. The value of w_T for a particular organ or tissue represents the fraction of detriment (*i.e.*, from cancer and hereditary effects) attributed to that organ or tissue when the whole body is irradiated uniformly. Tissue weighting factors are assigned for 12 tissues and organs and a remainder for assignment to other tissues and organs as necessary such that the sum of these factors equals one. The equivalent dose to a specific organ or tissue (H_T) is obtained by weighting the mean absorbed dose in a tissue or organ (see below) (D_T) by a radiation weighting factor (w_R) to allow for the relative biological effectiveness of the ionizing radiation or radiations of interest. Based on the radiation risks determined from epidemiological and animal studies, values of E are assigned as various effective dose limits (E_{limit}) for purposes of radiation protection.

With the development of advanced calculational techniques of interactions of radiations with matter (*e.g.*, Monte-Carlo radiation transport analysis), it is possible to estimate the relationship between air kerma and effective dose using conversion coefficients that are published in ICRU Report 57 (ICRU, 1998b). These calculations provide the effective dose per unit of air kerma ($E\,K_a^{-1}$) (in Sv Gy^{-1}) for monoenergetic photons in various geometries incident on an adult anthropomorphic computational model. The geometries published are anterior-posterior, posterior-anterior, right- and left-lateral, rotational (ROT) and isotropic (ISO). The last two geometries, ROT and ISO, are most applicable to this Report because individuals will be moving around when interacting with a treated patient. The average of values for $E\,K_a^{-1}$ for the energy range 0.05 to 1 MeV is 0.846 for ROT and 0.682 for ISO. The conversion equation (ICRU, 1998b) for effective dose (in sieverts) is:

$$E = K_a(E\,K_a^{-1}) = 0.00876\,X\,(E\,K_a^{-1}), \tag{A.2}$$

where $E\,K_a^{-1}$ is the effective dose per unit air-kerma conversion coefficient as a function of photon energy and radiation geometry. Then, for the two applicable geometries (ICRU, 1998b):

$$E_{ROT} = (0.00876\ X)\ 0.846 = 0.00741\ X, \qquad\qquad (A.3)$$

$$E_{ISO} = (0.00876\ X)\ 0.682 = 0.00597\ X. \qquad\qquad (A.4)$$

Alternatively, E_{ROT} and E_{ISO} can be obtained by dividing X by 135 and 168, respectively.

Both geometries are given for illustration purposes. For a specific situation, the applicable photon energy can be used and the appropriate geometry chosen. Thus, a conservatively safe assumption is that the measured or calculated value of K_a, determined directly or using the measured exposure X, will be an overestimate of the effective dose E for the exposed individual.

As a practical example, Sparks *et al*. (1998) have investigated the use of ^{131}I in radioimmunotherapy patients. Their Monte-Carlo analysis indicates that the numerical value for effective dose equivalent (the predecessor quantity to effective dose) at 1 m is only 62 % of the measured absorbed dose in air (D_a) at 1 m.

A.2 Exposed Groups and Dose Limits

In Report No. 37 and Commentary No. 11 (NCRP, 1970; 1995a), NCRP considered the radiation doses to family members and others in the vicinity of a patient treated with radiopharmaceutical therapy and brachytherapy. Those recommendations formed the basis of the recommendations of Regulatory Guide 8.39 (NRC, 1997) and its successor document, NUREG-1556 (NRC, 1997; 2005). A "family member" may be any person who spends a substantial amount of time in the company of the patient on a regular basis, providing support and comfort, and whom the patient considers a member of their "family," whether by birth, by marriage, or by virtue of a close, caring relationship (NCRP, 1995a). Members of a patient's family can and *should* be considered as distinct from members of the public in many respects, including the application of radiation protection standards. Standards for family members of radionuclide therapy patients *should not* be as restrictive as those for members of the public because family members receive benefits associated with treatment of the patient and they accept their radiation burden as explained by the treating physician.

Radionuclide therapies are generally employed no more than several times during a patient's lifetime, and family members of patients receiving such therapies *should*, therefore, be considered as being exposed infrequently, with a recommended annual effective dose limit (E_{limit}) of 5 mSv (NCRP, 1993b).[5] In addition, in

Commentary No. 11, NCRP recommended that an adult member of the patient's family be permitted to receive up to 50 mSv y^{-1} on the recommendation of the treating physician (NCRP, 1995a).[6] Although an endorsement of the 5 mSv y^{-1} limit specified in NRC's Regulatory Guide 8.39 (NRC, 1997) is not implied or intended, this value of the E_{limit} is used in the development of the analytical basis described in this Appendix.

A "member of the public" may be any individual who is not a patient undergoing treatment, is not a family member of such a patient, and is not an occupationally-exposed individual participating in the care and management of such a patient. Members of the public include other patients in the medical facility in which the patient may be confined, the patient's co-workers, and other individuals with no familial connection to the patient. Use of the 1 mSv y^{-1} limit for members of the public and for children and pregnant women in the patient's family is consistent with the limits recommended for these groups by NCRP (1995a). It should be noted that the foregoing limits are annual totals and, therefore, do not apply to individual treatments of a patient but collectively to all treatments a patient may receive in a given year (NCRP, 1993b; 1995a).

The practical requirement in protecting a person from the radiation emitted by a patient is to determine the effective dose, as discussed above, during the period of time when the exposure rate from the patient is significant. The effective dose then is the product of the effective dose rate and the period of exposure. Because the exposure rate from the patient is continuously decreasing with time from radioactive decay and from biological elimination of the radionuclide, the effective dose rate is also continuously decreasing and appropriate mathematical calculation is required as discussed in the analytical presentation that follows.

In 1996 NRC analyzed the practical consequences of a relaxation of the regulatory requirements for medical confinement of radionuclide therapy patients (NRC, 1997a). The conclusions of this analysis were that projected dose-based release criteria, in replacing the long-standing activity-based criteria, would not pose a significant radiation risk to the public and would result in outpatient

---

[5]Corresponds to the effective dose limit for infrequent exposures of the public recommended in NCRP Report No. 116 (NCRP, 1993b).

[6]NCRP Statement No. 10 (NCRP, 2004a) and NCRP Commentary No. 11 (NCRP, 1995a) recommend this upper limit for nonpregnant adults on recommendation of the treating physician provided these persons receive appropriate training and individual monitoring.

treatment of many radionuclide therapy patients who would other-wise require hospitalization. Shortly thereafter, NRC codified new release criteria described in Regulatory Guide 8.39 for radionuclide therapy patients (NRC, 1997b). A sizable literature rapidly emerged on their practical implementation. An algorithm was developed by Gates *et al.* (1998) and by Siegel (1998) for therapy of non-Hodgkin's B-cell lymphoma with ^{131}I-labeled anti-B1 mono-clonal antibody. The total-body clearance of this agent followed mono-exponential kinetics, that is, the total-body time-activity could be described mathematically by a single exponential term (Gates *et al.*, 1998; Siegel, 1998). With noted exceptions, such an approach had not appeared previously in the scientific literature (Barrington *et al.*, 1999; Cormack and Shearer, 1998). This new approach was expanded by Zanzonico *et al.* (2000) who presented a generalized algorithm for determining the time of release and the duration at home of post-release radiation precautions following radiopharmaceutical therapy. The E_{limit} for some groups used in the development of this algorithm differs from previous recommenda-tions of NCRP. For each type of group of exposed or potentially exposed individuals, the most conservatively safe (*i.e.*, the lowest) E_{limit} value stipulated or recommended has been used.

A.3 Occupancy Factors and Index Distances

Important in the estimation of effective dose are two interre-lated parameters: the occupancy factor and what has been termed the "index distance" (NRC, 2002). The occupancy factor (T_{r_j}) at an index distance, r_j, from a radioactive patient is the fraction of time an individual spends at the index distance from the patient such that $\sum_{j=1}^{m} T_{r_j} = 1$. This relation represents the sum over all index distances up to a maximal distance r_m from the patient. For every-day activities, the index distance is set at 1 m. The mean index dis-tance between sleeping partners and between a child and an individual holding the child is set at 0.3 m. Such index distances are, of course, difficult to establish precisely and are inevitably somewhat arbitrary, but the distances appear to be consistent with the limited anthropological data available (Culver and Dworkin, 1991; 1992; Hall, 1966; Siegel, 1998). However, the algorithm does not depend on any specific values of occupancy factors and index distances. The parameters shown in Table A.1 and the related equations that follow can be modified as deemed appropriate.

When not specifically in the company of the radioactive patient, an individual will be at distances well beyond the index distance of 1 m. Because of the rapid decrease in exposure rate with distance from the patient, for distances other than or farther from the radioactive patient than these specified index distances, the exposure rates may be considered negligibly small. Accordingly, in practice, distances other than the specified index distances and the associated occupancy factors shown in Table A.1 are not explicitly considered and, therefore, $\sum\limits_{j=1}^{m} T_{r_j} \neq 1$.

A.4 Operational Equations

The time-dependent effective dose rate at an index distance r_j from a patient containing activity may be approximated using the following equations (Zanzonico, 2000):[7]

TABLE A.1—*Occupancy factors, index distances, and effective dose limits.*

Group/Activity	Occupancy Factors	Index Distances (m)	Effective Dose Limits (mSv)
Members of patients' family:			
Nonsleeping partner/adult	0.25	1.0	5
Nonpregnant sleeping partner	0.33	0.3	5
Pregnant sleeping partner	0.33	0.3	1
Pregnant women/children	0.25	1.0	1/1
Child held by patient	0.20	0.3	1
Public: Co-worker	0.33	1.0	1

[7]Equations A.5 to A.12 have all been adapted from Zanzonico (2000).

$$\dot{E}(r_j, t) = \dot{K}_a(r_j, t)(E \, K_a^{-1}) \tag{A.5}$$

$$= \sum_{i=1}^{n} \dot{K}_a(r_j, 0)_i (E \, K_a^{-1}) e^{\frac{-0.693 t}{T_{e_i}}} ,$$

where:

$\dot{E}(r_j, t)$ = effective dose rate (mSv h⁻¹) at an index distance r_j (meters) from the patient at time t post-administration (days)

$\dot{K}_a(r_j, t)$ = air kerma rate (Gy h⁻¹) at an index distance r_j (meters) from the patient at time t post-administration (days)

$E \, K_a^{-1}$ = effective dose per unit air kerma conversion coefficient (Sv Gy⁻¹)

$\dot{K}_a(r_j, 0)_i$ = zero-time intercept of exponential component i of the time-dependent air kerma rate measured at an index distance r_j (meters) from the patient

T_{e_i} = effective half-life (days) of the nondecay corrected total-body activity for compartment i of a multi-exponential function

n = number of exponential components required to describe the time-dependent total-body activity

Implicit in Equation A.5 is the overestimation approximately by a factor of two, previously described, when using the air kerma rate that is actually measured in practice and that applies throughout the analysis that follows. Also, implicit in Equation A.5 is the assumption that the time-dependent total-body activity follows a multi-exponential function:

$$A(t) = A(0) \sum_{i=1}^{n} F_i e^{\frac{-0.693 t}{T_{e_i}}} , \tag{A.6}$$

where:

$A(t)$ = total-body activity (becquerels) at time t post-administration (days)

F_i = zero-time intercept of exponential component i of the total-body activity expressed as a fraction of the administered activity such that $\sum_{i=1}^{n} F_i = 1$

The foregoing activities are decay corrected, that is, the activity is corrected for radioactive decay back to the time of administration. In principle, each of the exponential components represents a metabolic compartment and its effective half-life is related to the rate of clearance of activity from that compartment.

In addition, implicit in these equations is the assumption that activity is being continuously eliminated from the patient's body from the time of administration. Of course, no activity is biologically eliminated from the body before the patient's first void or defecation post-therapy. Within these first several hours post-therapy, the only means of elimination of activity is physical decay. Various authors account for this by appending an effective dose contribution term with an effective half-life equal to the particular radionuclide's physical half-life (Gates et al., 1998; NRC, 2002; Siegel, 1998). The duration of time during which an effective half-life is equal to the radionuclide's physical half-life is taken as 8 h for orally administered radiopharmaceuticals such as ^{131}I-labeled sodium iodide but only 3 h for intravenously administered radiopharmaceuticals such as ^{131}I anti-B1 monoclonal antibody (Gates et al., 1998; NRC, 2005; Siegel, 1998). The 8 h period may be overly conservative (in the safe direction), because gastric emptying and overall gastrointestinal elimination of orally administered radiopharmaceuticals in liquid form will likely occur earlier than 8 h. An alternative approach, implicitly represented in the equations above, is that the patient remains in the hospital until the first post-therapy void/defecation or for some designated time by which the activity in the stomach following oral administration would have dramatically decreased. The decision as to choice of this time is somewhat arbitrary, but a minimal time of 2 h would seem prudent. This approach may require an appropriately designed room in which to house the radioactive patient immediately following administration of the therapeutic activity. This room may have to be a dedicated facility depending on the patient volume. The room *should* be supplied with portable or fixed shielding to reduce the dose levels in the surrounding areas to public levels. Consideration *should* be given to shielding of waste collection cans and areas for performing release surveys. Special design considerations *should* be reviewed with a qualified medical physicist.

The values of the parameters, F_i and T_{e_i}, of the multi-exponential function in Equation A.6 may be obtained from sources in the pertinent scientific literature or, preferably, be determined empirically for individual patients by performing serial measurements of the total-body activity following a pretherapy tracer administration of the therapeutic radiopharmaceutical and mono-

or multi-exponential curve-fitting of the resulting time-activity data (Zanzonico, 1995). Following determination of the F_i and T_{e_i}, Equation A.5 may then be rewritten as:

$$\dot{E}(r_j, t) = \dot{K}_a(r_j, 0)(E K_a^{-1}) \sum_{i=1}^{n} F_i e^{\frac{-0.693t}{T_{e_i}}}. \tag{A.7}$$

Thus, the effective dose at an index distance r_j from a radioactive patient from time t_1 to time t_2 post-administration is given by the following equation as:

$$E(r_j)_{t_1 \rightarrow t_2} = 24 \, T_{r_j} \dot{K}_a(r_j, 0)(E K_a^{-1}) \sum_{i=1}^{n} \int_{t_1}^{t_2} F_i e^{\frac{-0.693t}{T_{e_i}}} dt, \tag{A.8}$$

where:

$E(r_j)_{t_1 \rightarrow t_2}$ = effective dose (millisieverts) at an index distance r_j from the patient from time t_1 to time t_2 post-administration (days)

$E K_a^{-1}$ = effective dose per unit air kerma conversion coefficient (Sv Gy^{-1})

T_{r_j} = occupancy factor for an individual at a distance r_j (meters) from a radioactive patient

24 = factor for conversion of time in days to time in hours

Equation A.8 may be generalized to yield the effective dose from a radioactive patient from time t_1 to time t_2 ($E_{t_1 \rightarrow t_2}$) post-administration including all possible occupancy factors as:

$$E_{t_1 \rightarrow t_2} = 24 \sum_{j=1}^{m} T_{r_j} \dot{K}_a(r_j, 0)(E K_a^{-1}) \sum_{i=1}^{n} \int_{t_1}^{t_2} F_i e^{\frac{-0.693t}{T_{e_i}}} dt. \tag{A.9}$$

By substituting $t_1 = 0$ and $t_2 = $ into Equation A.9 and evaluating the resulting definite integral[8] the effective dose from the patient over all time can be obtained as:

[8]Note that $\sum_{i=1}^{n} \int_{t_1}^{t_2} F_i e^{\frac{-0.693t}{T_{e_i}}} dt = 1.44 \sum_{i=1}^{n} F_i T_{e_i}$ where the factor 1.44 = 1/0.693.

$$E = 24 \sum_{\varphi = 1}^{m} T_{r_j} \dot{K}_a(r_j, 0)(E \, K_a^{-1}) \, 1.44 \sum_{i = 1}^{n} F_i \, T_{e_i} \qquad (A.10)$$

$$= 24 \, \tau \sum_{j = 1}^{m} \dot{K}_a(r_j, 0)(E \, K_a^{-1}) \, T_{r_j},$$

where:

τ =   the residence time (days) of activity in the patient

$$= 1.44 \sum_{i = 1}^{n} F_i \, T_{e_i}$$

When the patient is to be released from medical confinement, the effective dose for any person associated with the patient arising from the air kerma rate of such a patient at the release time (t_{release}), *shall not* exceed the applicable dose limit. The time of release [($t_{\text{release}})_{\text{limit}}$], then becomes the controlling factor in determining the effective dose at time of release [$E(t_{\text{release}})_{\text{limit}}$], that is to be compared to the effective dose limit (E_{limit}). Thus, by substituting $t_1 = (t_{\text{release}})_{\text{limit}}$ and $t_2 = \infty$, Equation A.9 becomes:

$$E_{\text{limit}} = 34.6 \sum_{j = 1}^{m} T_{r_j} \dot{K}_a(r_j, 0)(E \, K_a^{-1}) \sum_{i = 1}^{n} T_{e_i} \, F_i e^{\frac{-0.693(t_{\text{release}})_{\text{limit}}}{T_{e_i}}} \qquad (A.11)$$

for the whole period after release, where 34.6 = 1.44 × 24, a factor for calculating residence time (τ) (hours), from the fractional zero-time intercepts (F_i), and the effective half-lives (T_{e_i}) (days).

Equation A.11 cannot be solved analytically for the parameter ($t_{\text{release}})_{\text{limit}}$, that is, Equation A.11 cannot be solved to provide an explicit formula for the parameter ($t_{\text{release}})_{\text{limit}}$ for a multi-exponential total-body time-activity function (Cormack, 1998). However, the time post-administration for release of the patient from medical confinement, $t_1 = (t_{\text{release}})_{\text{limit}}$, and the duration of various radiation precautions may be determined "iteratively" from Equation A.11. If the effective dose (E) at an index distance of 1 m from the radiopharmaceutical therapy or brachytherapy patient as given by Equation A.11 does not exceed the effective dose limit of 5 mSv, the patient may be released after administration of the therapeutic radiopharmaceutical or implant following the restrictions on a first void and time restrictions as discussed previously. If, however, E at an index distance of 1 m from the radiopharmaceutical therapy or brachytherapy patient as given by Equation A.11 does exceed the effective dose limit of 5 mSv, possible values of the time post-administration of release of the patient from medical confinement $[(t_{release})_{0.5\ cSv}]$ may be substituted into the right side of Equation A.11. Beginning with a time of 1 d and substituting time values in 1 d increments, the smallest time value (1 d, 2 d, 3 d...) that yields an effective dose by Equation A.11 equal to or less than the dose limit is the time post-administration of release of the patient from medical confinement $[(t_{release})_{limit}]$. Similarly, the duration in terms of times post-administration of the post-release radiation precautions [*i.e.*, *not* working $(t_{no\ work})$, avoiding pregnant women and children (t_{avoid}), limiting holding of children $(t_{no\ hold})$, and sleeping partners *not* sleeping together $(t_{sleep\ apart})$] may be determined with Equation A.11 by substituting the dose limits applicable to the respective groups and the corresponding index distances (r_j), occupancy factors (T_{r_j}), and measured zero-time air kerma rates $[\dot{K}(r_j, 0)]$. Increments shorter than 1 d may be used for this calculation. Depending on the group(s) of interest, which in turn depends on the circumstances of the individual patient, the pertinent values of the effective-dose limits, the index distances (r_j) and the occupancy factors (T_{r_j}) will vary and the exact form of Equation A.11 will, therefore, vary as well. It can be useful to calculate these times using a computerized spreadsheet program.

For a therapeutic radiopharmaceutical for which the time-dependent total-body activity follows a mono-exponential function (*i.e.*, in Equation A.5, $n = 1$) Equation A.11 can be expressed as:

$$E_{limit} = 34.6 \sum_{j=1}^{m} T_{r_j} \dot{K}_a(r_j, 0)(E\ K_a^{-1})\ T_e\ e^{\dfrac{-0.693(t_{release})_{limit}}{T_e}}, \quad (A.12)$$

where:

T_e = effective half-life of the nondecay-corrected total-body activity for a single exponential function

Mono-exponential total-body time-activity functions apply, at least approximately, to many therapeutic radiopharmaceuticals. In contrast to Equation A.11, Equation A.12 can be solved explicitly for $(t_{release})_{limit}$, the time of release from medical confinement following radionuclide treatment.

Use of the appropriate group-dependent effective-dose limits, index distances (r_j), and occupancy factors (T_{r_j}), the practical forms of Equation A.11 (*i.e.*, the so-called "general operational equations" for multi-exponential clearance) can be used to determine the times post-radiopharmaceutical treatment for release from medical confinement $[t(_{release})_{limit}]$, *not* working $(t_{no\ work})$, avoiding pregnant women and children (t_{avoid}), limiting holding of children $(t_{no\ hold})$, and sleeping partners *not* sleeping together $(t_{sleep\ apart})$ (Table A.2).

In addition, Equation A.12 has been solved explicitly, yielding the so-called "special operational equations" for the corresponding times post-radiopharmaceutical treatment for mono-exponential clearance (Table A.3).

In Tables A.2 and A.3, the second main entry "Members of Patients Family" has two subentries: (1) "all activities except sleeping with the patient" and (2) "sleeping with the patient." The patient then has a choice that must be made before being released so that the dose calculation can be made and the results entered in the instruction sheets of Appendix B. Both Options 1 and 2 can be analyzed and the sums of the two associated doses *shall not* exceed the dose limit of 5 mSv. Alternatively, the patient can choose to use the longer time, $t_{release}$ or $t_{sleep\ apart}$, resulting from each of the options to meet the dose limit.

If it is deemed appropriate by the physician in consultation with the RSO that a patient is not suitable for release following same-day treatment, then the patient *should* be admitted to the medical facility (Section 3). In these cases, the exposure-rate criteria for release *should* be consistent with both licensing restrictions and regulatory dose limits.

TABLE A.2—*General operational equations for multi-exponential retention of therapeutic radiopharmaceuticals.*[a] Determination of time post-radiopharmaceutical treatment of release from medical confinement [$(t_{release})_{limit}$], of *not* working ($t_{no\ work}$), of avoiding pregnant women and children (t_{avoid}), of limiting holding of children ($t_{no\ hold}$), and of sleeping partners *not* sleeping together ($t_{sleep\ apart}$).

Group/Activity	Index Distance (m)	Occupancy Factor	Effective-Dose Limit (cSv)	Operational Equation for Determining Specified Time (d)[a]
Nonpregnant Adult				
Members of patient's family				
Nonsleeping partner	1	0.25	0.5	$0.5 = 8.64\,\dot{K}_a(1,0)(E\,K_a^{-1}) \sum_{i=1}^{n} T_{e_i} F_i e^{\dfrac{-0.693(t_{release})_{0.5\,cSv}}{T_{e_i}}}$
Sleeping partner				
All activities *except* sleeping with patient	1	0.25		$0.5 = 8.64\,\dot{K}_a(1,0)(E\,K_a^{-1}) \sum_{i=1}^{n} T_{e_i} F_i e^{\dfrac{-0.693(t_{release})_{0.5\,cSv}}{T_{e_i}}}$
plus/or[b]			0.5	plus/or
Sleeping with patient	0.3	0.33		$0.5 = 11.4\,\dot{K}_a(0.3,0)(E\,K_a^{-1}) \sum_{i=1}^{n} T_{e_i} F_i e^{\dfrac{-0.693(t_{sleep\ apart})}{T_{e_i}}}$

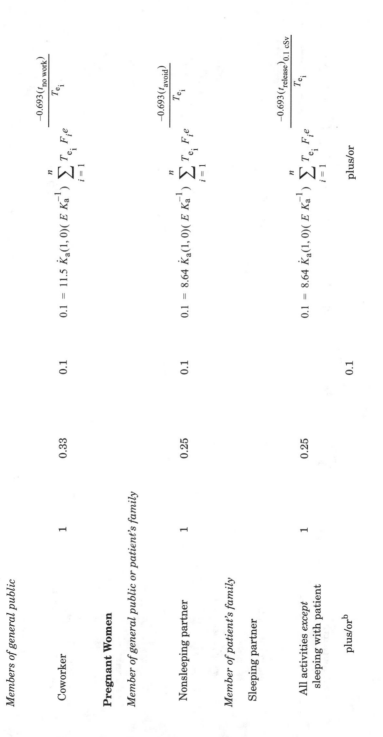

Members of general public

Coworker 1 0.33 0.1

$$0.1 = 11.5\,\dot{K}_a(1,0)(E\,K_a^{-1}) \sum_{i=1}^{n} T_{e_i} F_i\, e^{\frac{-0.693(t_{\text{no work}})}{T_{e_i}}}$$

Pregnant Women

Member of general public or patient's family

Nonsleeping partner 1 0.25 0.1

$$0.1 = 8.64\,\dot{K}_a(1,0)(E\,K_a^{-1}) \sum_{i=1}^{n} T_{e_i} F_i\, e^{\frac{-0.693(t_{\text{avoid}})}{T_{e_i}}}$$

Member of patient's family

Sleeping partner

All activities *except* sleeping with patient 1 0.25 0.1

$$0.1 = 8.64\,\dot{K}_a(1,0)(E\,K_a^{-1}) \sum_{i=1}^{n} T_{e_i} F_i\, e^{\frac{-0.693(t_{\text{release}})_{0.1\,\text{cSv}}}{T_{e_i}}}$$

plus/or

plus/or[b] 0.1

TABLE A.2—(continued).

Group/Activity	Index Distance (m)	Occupancy Factor	Effective-Dose Limit (cSv)	Operational Equation for Determining Specified Time (d)[a]
Sleeping with patient	0.3	0.33		$0.1 = 11.4 \, \dot{K}_a(0.3, 0)(E \, K_a^{-1}) \sum_{i=1}^{n} T_{e_i} F_i e^{\frac{-0.693(t_{\text{sleep apart}})}{T_{e_i}}}$
Members of general public				
Coworker	1	0.33	0.1	$0.1 = 11.5 \, \dot{K}_a(1, 0)(E \, K_a^{-1}) \sum_{i=1}^{n} T_{e_i} F_i e^{\frac{-0.693(t_{\text{no work}})}{T_{e_i}}}$
Children				
All activities *except* patient holding child	1	0.25	0.1	$0.1 = 8.64 \, \dot{K}_a(1, 0)(E \, K_a^{-1}) \sum_{i=1}^{n} T_{e_i} F_i e^{\frac{-0.693(t_{\text{release}})}{T_{e_i}}}$
plus/or[b]				plus/or

| Patient holding child | 0.3 | 0.2 | $0.1 = 7.2\,\dot{K}_a(0.3, 0)(E\,K_a^{-1})\displaystyle\sum_{i=1}^{n} T_{e_i}\,F_i\,e^{\dfrac{-0.693(t_{no\ hold})}{T_{e_i}}}$ |

[a]Equations adapted from Zanzonico (2000).
[b]The "plus/or" indicates two choices in meeting the dose limit. In one, the sums of the doses from the two equations for the same times or different times *shall not* exceed the dose limit. Alternatively, the patient can choose the longest time, $t_{release}$ or t_{sleep} apart, resulting from each of the options to meet the dose limit.

TABLE A.3—*Special operational equations for mono-exponential retention of therapeutic radiopharmaceuticals.*[a]
Determination of time post-radiopharmaceutical treatment of release from medical confinement [$(t_{release})_{limit}$], of not working ($t_{no\ work}$), of avoiding pregnant women and children (t_{avoid}) of limiting holding of children ($t_{no\ hold}$), and of sleeping partners not sleeping together ($t_{sleep\ apart}$).

Group/Activity	Index Distance (m)	Occupancy Factor	Effective-Dose Limit (cSv)	Operational Equation for Determining Specified Time (d)[a]
Nonpregnant Adult				
Members of patient's family				
Nonsleeping partner	1	0.25	0.5	$(t_{release})_{0.5\ cSv} = 1.44\ T_e\ \ln[1.72\ \dot{K}_a(1,0)(E\ K_a^{-1})T_e]$
Sleeping partner				
All activities *except* sleeping with patient	1	0.25		
plus/or[b,c]			0.5	$t_{sleep\ apart} = 1.44\ T_e\ \ln\left[\dfrac{\dfrac{-0.693(t_{release})_{0.5\ cSv}}{T_e}}{\dfrac{0.029}{T_e} - 0.33\ \dot{K}_a(1,0)(E\ K_a^{-1})e}\right]$
Sleeping with patient	0.3	0.33		

Members of general public

Coworker	1	0.33	0.1	$t_{\text{no work}} = 1.44\, T_e \ln[86.4\, \dot{K}_a(1,\,0)(E\,K_a^{-1})T_e]$

Pregnant Women

Members of general public or patient's family

| Nonsleeping partner | 1 | 0.25 | 0.1 | $t_{\text{avoid}} = 1.44\, T_e \ln[86.4\, \dot{K}_a(1,\,0)(E\,K_a^{-1})T_e]$ |

Member of patient's family

Sleeping partner

| All activities *except* sleeping with patient | 1 | 0.25 | 0.1 | |

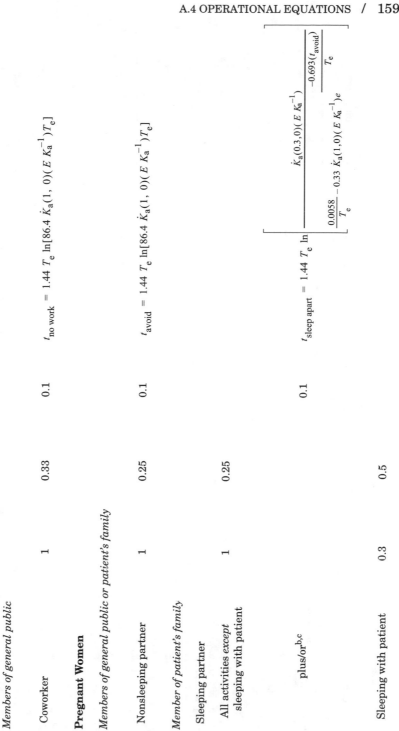

$$t_{\text{sleep apart}} = 1.44\, T_e\, \ln\left[\frac{\dfrac{0.0058}{T_e} - 0.33\,\dot{K}_a(1,0)(E\,K_a^{-1})e^{\frac{-0.693(t_{\text{avoid}})}{T_e}}}{\dot{K}_a(0.3,0)(E\,K_a^{-1})}\right]$$

plus/or[b,c]

| Sleeping with patient | 0.3 | 0.5 | |

TABLE A.3—(continued).

Group/Activity	Index Distance (m)	Occupancy Factor	Effective-Dose Limit (cSv)	Operational Equation for Determining Specified Time (d)[a]
Members of general public				
Coworker	1	0.33	0.1	$t_{\text{no work}} = 1.44\, T_e\, \ln[86.4\, \dot{K}_a(1,\,0)(E\, K_a^{-1})T_e]$
Children				
All activities *except* patient holding child	1	0.25	0.1	
plus/or[b,c]				$t_{\text{no hold}} = 1.44\, T_e\, \ln\left[\dfrac{\dot{K}_a(0.3,\,0)(E\, K_a^{-1})}{\dfrac{0.014}{T_e} - 1.2\, \dot{K}_a(1,\,0)(E\, K_a^{-1})e^{\frac{-0.693(t_{\text{avoid}})}{T_e}}}\right]$
Patient holding child	0.3	0.2		

[a]Equations adapted from Zanzonico (2000).

[b]The "plus/or" indicates two choices in meeting the dose limit. In one, the sums of the doses from the two equations for the same times or different times must not exceed the dose limit. Alternatively, the patient can choose the longest time, t_{release} or t_{sleep} apart, resulting from each of the options to meet the dose limit.

[c]For mono-exponential retention, only one equation applies in the dose calculation for each subentry, but different values are entered for index distance and occupancy factor.

Appendix B

Examples of the Application of the Operational Equations Given in Appendix A

To facilitate the understanding of the operational equations presented in Appendix A, several examples illustrating the practical application of these equations have been formulated and are presented in this Appendix.[9] The spreadsheets[10] for the examples that follow include pertinent numerical data and dosimetry results based on all the assumptions and equations presented in Appendix A. These illustrations are intended as examples only and *should* not be taken to imply that the treatments described are

---

[9]Although SI units are used in the Report, conventional units are used in certain instances of this Appendix to enhance the practical usability of the information presented.

[10]The spreadsheet file used for calculating the numerical values in the Appendix B examples is provided as professional information for educational purposes only. The spreadsheet file is a nonvalidated calculation tool for which there is absolutely no guarantee or warranty of fitness for a particular purpose or any purpose expressed or implied. Any user of information contained herein assumes any and all responsibility and liability for use of the information including any misunderstanding, misuse or misapplication of the information. Any use of this spreadsheet file is "as is" and should only follow the user's independent confirmation that it produces valid results for the user before results are used for any purpose whatsoever. In no event *shall* the authors of the NCRP Report or NCRP itself be liable for any incorrect or invalid results that are obtained by any use of this spreadsheet file nor *shall* the authors or NCRP be liable for any loss of data, or profits or special, incidental, indirect or consequential damages arising out of or in connection with the use or performance of this spreadsheet file.

either directly or indirectly applicable to any patient. The decision as to the amount of activity to administer to a particular patient remains the responsibility of the prescribing physician.

In the following examples, note that patients can be released from the hospital on the day of treatment or 1 or 2 d later. However, there can be sufficient activity in the patients with half-lives long enough to require the observance for many days of the instructions to be performed after release, especially at home (*i.e.*, the duration for the instructions and actions can be extended over a period of time and the period will depend on the particular treatment situation).

Patients *should* be asked to acknowledge the instructions provided by the facility, preferably in writing (*e.g.*, by signing a release form of the type suggested at the end of the instructions for each example). Also the patients *should* be given a copy of the instructions, including the copy of the release form.

B.1 Example 1: Metastatic Thyroid Cancer

In Example 1, a post-thyroidectomy and post-radioiodine ablation patient with metastatic thyroid cancer has been treated with an administered activity of 6,475 MBq (175 mCi) of ^{131}I as sodium iodide. Based on kinetic measurements of a pretherapy administration of a 74 MBq (2 mCi) ^{131}I sodium-iodide tracer, this patient was found to exhibit a bi-phasic (bi-exponential) retention function (*i.e.*, total-body time-activity function), eliminating 95 % of the administered activity with an effective half-life of 0.32 d and the remaining 5 % with an effective half-time of 5.8 d, yielding an ^{131}I "residence time" of 0.86 d = 20.5 h. In the literature on internal radionuclide dosimetry, the quantity cumulated activity in an organ is sometimes used in place of the quantity residence time (τ), equivalent to the cumulated activity ($\tilde{A}$) per unit administered activity (AA):

$$\tau = \frac{\tilde{A}}{AA} = 1.44 \sum_i \frac{A_i}{AA} T_{e_i} = 1.44 \sum_i F_i T_{e_i} \qquad (B.1)$$

where:

T_{e_i} = effective half-life

F_i = fraction of the administered activity at time $t = 0$ for the ith exponential component of the time-activity function in the organ

Therefore, $\tilde{A} = AA\tau$ is units of s^{-1}. Immediately following administration of the 74 MBq (2 mCi) tracer, exposure rates were measured with a survey meter, yielding 0.26 and 3 mR h^{-1} at 1 and 0.3 m, respectively.

Accordingly, because all of the Column 1 values in the spreadsheet are <5 mSv this patient could be released on the same day the treatment was administered. However, the patient *should* avoid holding small children for >10 min d^{-1} for 21 d post-treatment, and only if the patient avoided the children altogether during the first day after treatment when the patient was the most radioactive and, therefore, producing the highest exposure rate. This restriction is necessitated by the fact that the values in the "1 d" subcolumn in Column 6 do not decrease to <1 mSv until after day 21 post-treatment. As indicated in the other subcolumns in Column 6, this "child-avoidance" period is shortened somewhat if the patient avoided children altogether for longer than 1 d immediately post-treatment. Conversely, if the patient did not avoid children during that first day post-treatment, the subsequent "child-avoidance period is much longer, as the values in the "0 d" subcolumn in Column 6 do not decrease to <1 mSv even up to day 40 post-treatment.

Because all of the Column 4 values after the first day post-treatment are <1 mSv, the patient can return to work on day two post-treatment. Likewise, the general radiation precautions at home need to be observed only for the first day post-treatment subject to the other dose restrictions. On the other hand, the patient *should not* sleep in the same bed with a sleeping partner until 7 d after treatment, as the values in the "0 d" subcolumn in Column 3 do not decrease to <5 mSv until day seven post-treatment. However, if the patient's sleeping partner is pregnant, her dose limit is lowered to 1 mSv and the patient *should*, therefore, not sleep in the same bed until 24 d after treatment, and only if he avoided his sleeping partner altogether during the first day after administration of the radiopharmaceutical therapy, as the values in the "1 d" subcolumn in Column 3 do not decrease to <1 mSv until after 24 d post-treatment.

The spreadsheet and instructions for this patient are on the following five pages (Zanzonico *et al.*, 2000).

Example 1 Spreadsheet

Times Post-Radionuclide Treatment of Release from Medical Confinement ($(t_{release})_{limd}$), of Not Working ($t_{no\ work}$), of Avoiding Pregnant Women and Children (t_{avoid}), of Limited Holding of Children ($t_{no\ hold}$), and of Sleeping Partners Not Sleeping Together ($t_{sleep\ apart}$)

Patient's Name: John Q. Patient
Patient's Number: 111-11-111
Therapeutic Radionuclide: Iodine-131
Therapeutic Radiopharmaceutical: Sodium Iodide
Disease / Condition: Metastatic thyroid cancer

Administered activity: 6,475 MBq
175 mCi
Date of Treatment: January 1, 1999
Time of Treatment: 6:00 AM

Parameters of Total-Body Time-Activity Function

F1	0.95	
Te1	0.32	d
F2	0.05	
Te2	5.8	d
F3		
Te3		d

Residence time (τ): 0.86 d 20.5 h

Parameters for up to three exponential components may be entered. If fewer than three apply, leave the cells for the parameters for the un-needed component(s) blank

Assumed Occupancy Factors

Family member	1 m =	0.25
Sleeping partner	0.3 m =	0.33
Coworker	1 m =	0.33
Held child*	0.3 m =	0.2

* Baby, toddler, or other child young enough to be regularly held by a care giver.
** Divide by 100 to obtain results in mSv h⁻¹ or mSv.

Measured Zero-Time Exposure Rates (mR h⁻¹)**

	at 1 m from upright patient	at 0.3 m from supine patient
per mCi	0.13	1.50
Total	23	263

Color Code for Tabulated Values Below

Gray	Activity NOT permitted Effective dose exceeds limit
White	Activity permitted Effective dose does NOT exceed limit

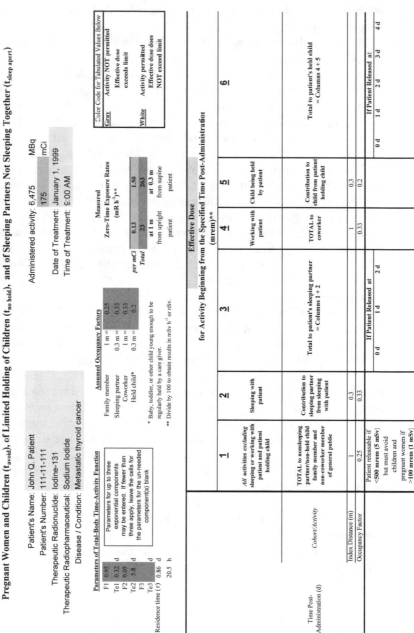

Effective Dose

for Activity Beginning from the Specified Time Post-Administration (mrem)**

Time Post-Administration (d)	Cohort/Activity	1 — All activities excluding sleeping or working with patient and patient holding child	2 — Sleeping with patient	3 — Total to patient's sleeping partner = Columns 1 + 2	4 — Working with patient	5 — Child being held by patient	6 — Total to patient's held child = Columns 4 + 5
		TOTAL to nonsleeping partner/non-held child family member and non-coworker member of general public	Contribution to sleeping partner from sleeping with patient		TOTAL to coworker	Contribution to child from patient holding child	
	Index Distance (m)	1	0.3		1	0.3	
	Occupancy Factor	0.25	0.33		0.33	0.2	
	Patient releasable if <500 mrem (5 mSv) but must avoid children and pregnant women if >100 mrem (1 mSv)			If Patient Released at 0 d 1 d 2 d			If Patient Released at 0 d 1 d 2 d 3 d 4 d

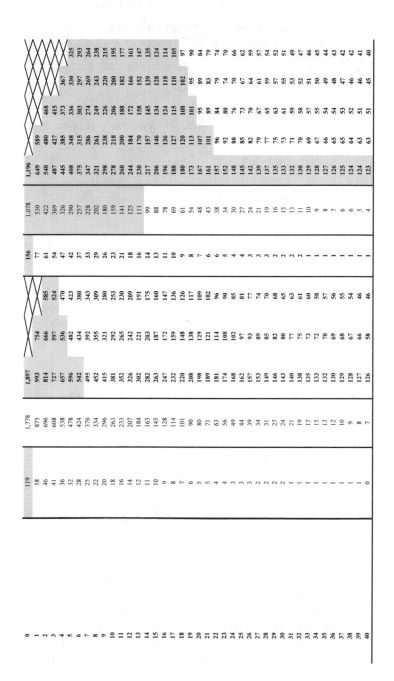

Example 1: Instruction Sheets

Radiation Safety Precautions for Radiopharmaceutical Therapy Patients

Note: Please carefully read and follow the instructions in this document.

If you or your health care provider have any questions or concerns regarding the radionuclide therapy you have received, please contact:

Dr. J. Smith
_____
Nuclear Medicine Attending Physician

at   (111) 222-3333
_____
Telephone Number

or   0000
_____
Emergency or Pager Telephone Number

Patient __John Q. Patient__ , Medical Record Number __111-11-111__ , received a therapeutic dose of __6.475 MBq (175 mCi)__ of __Iodine-131 Sodium Iodide__ at __General Hospital__ on __January 1, 2004__ at __9:00 am__ and *should* observe the following radiation safety precautions at home as follows.

- ☐   Avoid close contact [less than 1 meter (3 feet) away from] with pregnant women and children until __1 day__ after the administration of the radionuclide therapy.

- ☐   Do not hold or embrace children for more than 10 minutes a day until __21 days__ after the day your radionuclide therapy was administered. *This requires that you avoid contact with these children altogether during your* __first day__ *after the day your radionuclide therapy was administered.*

- ☐   Unless you work alone (for example, driving a truck), do not return to work until __1 day__ after the day your radionuclide therapy was administered.

- ☐   Do not sleep in the same bed with your sleeping partner until __7 days__ after the day your radionuclide therapy was administered.

- ☐   However, if your sleeping partner is pregnant, do not sleep in the same bed with your sleeping partner until __24 days__ after the day your radionuclide therapy was administered. This requires that you avoid contact with your pregnant sleeping partner *altogether* during your __first day__ after the day your radionuclide therapy was administered.

Patient: **Patient, John Q.**

MRN: **111-11-111**

In addition, the following precautions *should* be observed until 1 day after the administration of your radiopharmaceutical therapy.

- To the extent that is *reasonable*, generally try to remain as far away from individuals around you as possible.
- After using the toilet, flush twice and, as usual, wash your hands. If possible, use paper towels to dry your hands and dispose the paper toweling in the trash.
- You *should* otherwise observe good personal hygiene and may shower, bathe, shave, etc. as you normally would, rinsing the shower stall, tub or sink thoroughly after use.
- Wipe up any spills of urine, saliva and/or mucus with tissues or a small amount of disposable (*i.e.*, flushable) paper toweling, and dispose of the tissue or toweling down the toilet.
- Use nondisposable plates, bowls, spoons, knives, forks and cups. If possible, you *should* wash plates, bowls, spoons, knives, forks and cups which you use, using a separate sponge or wash cloth from that used by the rest of your household. Rinse the sink thoroughly after use, wipe the fixtures with paper towels, and dispose of the paper toweling in the trash.
- If you use a dishwasher, wash your plates, bowls, spoons, knives, forks and cups separately from those of the rest of your household.
- Use the same set of plates, bowls, spoons, knives and forks for 1 day after your radionuclide therapy.
- Store and launder your soiled/used clothing and bed linens separately from those of the rest of your household, running the rinse cycle two times at the completion of machine laundering.
- Do not share food or drinks with anyone.
- After using the telephone, wipe the receiver (especially the mouth piece) with paper towels, and dispose the paper toweling in the trash.

Signature Section (example release form)

I have read this form and all of my questions have been answered. By signing below, I acknowledge that I have read and accept all of the information above.

_____

Signature of patient or personal representative

_____

Print name of patient or personal representative

_____

Date

_____

Relation of personal representative to patient

B.2 Example 2: Hyperthyroidism

In Example 2, a hyperthyroid (Graves disease) patient was treated with an administered activity of 370 MBq (10 mCi) of ^{131}I as sodium iodide. Based on published kinetic data for ^{131}I sodium iodide administered to such patients as well as data from the 24 h thyroid uptake measurement for a 370 kBq (10 μCi) pretherapy tracer administered to this patient, a bi-phasic (bi-exponential) total-body clearance was projected, with elimination of 60 and 40 % of the administered activity with effective *half-lives* of 0.32 and 7 d, respectively, yielding an ^{131}I residence time of 4.31 d (103 h). In addition, survey meter measurements immediately following the therapeutic administration yielded exposure rates of 2.4 and 24 mR h^{-1} at 1 and 0.3 m, respectively.

Accordingly, because all of the Column 1 values in the spreadsheet are <5 mSv, this patient can be released on the same day the treatment was administered, because all of these values were actually <1 mSv, the patient need not avoid normal social interactions with children or pregnant women. However, the patient *should* avoid holding small children for >10 min d^{-1} for 24 d after being treated; necessitated by the fact that the values in the "1 d" subcolumn in Column 6 do not decrease to <1 mSv until after day 24 post-treatment.

Because all of the Column 4 values are <1 mSv, the patient can return to work immediately. Likewise, subject to the other dose restrictions, general radiation precautions at home are not actually required. Nonetheless, it would be prudent to advise the patient to observe such precautions for at least the first day post-treatment. On the other hand, the patient *should not* sleep in the same bed with a sleeping partner until 6 d after treatment, as the values in the "0 d" subcolumn in Column 3 do not decrease to <5 mSv (500 mrem) until day five post-treatment. However, if the patient's sleeping partner is pregnant, her dose limit is lowered to 1 mSv and the patient *should*, therefore, not sleep in the same bed until 29 d after treatment, as the values in the "0 d" subcolumn in Column 3 do not decrease to <1 mSv until after 29 d post-treatment.

The spreadsheet and instructions for this patient are on the following five pages (Zanzonico *et al.*, 2000).

Example 2 Spreadsheet

Times Post-Radionuclide Treatment of Release from Medical Confinement [($t_{release}$)$_{limit}$)], of Not Working ($t_{no\ work}$), of Avoiding Pregnant Women and Children (t_{avoid}), of Limited Holding of Children ($t_{no\ hold}$), and of Sleeping Partners Not Sleeping Together ($t_{sleep\ apart}$)

Patient's Name: Jane Q. Patient
Patient's Number: 222-22-222
Therapeutic Radionuclide: Iodine-131
Therapeutic Radiopharmaceutical: Sodium Iodide
Disease / Condition: Graves disease

Administered activity: 370 MBq
10 mCi
Date of Treatment: January 1, 2000
Time of Treatment: 9:00 AM

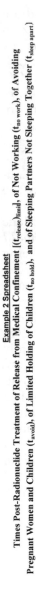

Parameters of Total-Body Time-Activity Function

F1	0.6		Parameters for up to three
Te1	0.32	d	exponential components
F2	0.4		may be entered. If fewer than
Te2	7	d	three apply, leave the cells for
F3			the parameters for the un-needed
Te3		d	component(s) blank
Residence time (τ)	4.31	d	
	103.4 h		

Assumed Occupancy Factors

Family member	1 m =	0.25
Sleeping partner	0.3 m =	0.33
Coworker	1 m =	0.33
Held child*	0.3 m =	0.2

* Baby, toddler, or other child young enough to be regularly held by a care giver.
** Divide by 100 to obtain results in mSv h⁻¹ or mSv.

Measured
Zero-Time Exposure Rates (mR h⁻¹)

	at 1 m from upright patient	at 0.3 m from supine patient
per mCi	0.24	2.4
Total	2.4	24

Color Code for Tabulated Values Below

| Gray | Activity NOT permitted | Effective dose exceeds limit |
| White | Activity permitted | Effective d+M32 NOT exceed limit |

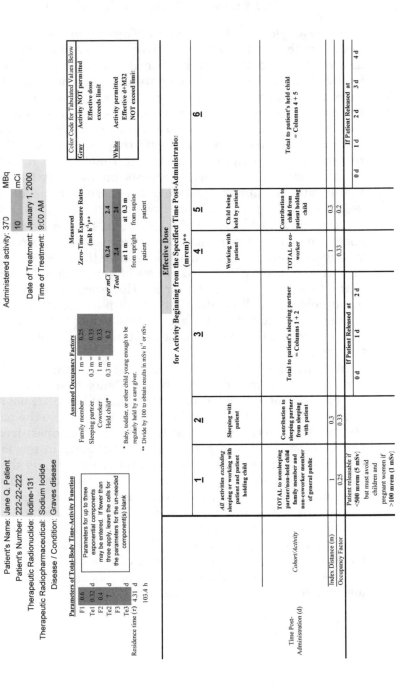

Effective Dose for Activity Beginning from the Specified Time Post-Administration (mrem)**

	1	2	3	4	5	6
Cohort/Activity	All activities *excluding* sleeping or working with patient and patient holding child	Sleeping with patient	Total to patient's sleeping partner = Columns 1 + 2	Working with patient	Child being held by patient	Total to patient's held child = Columns 4 + 5
	TOTAL to nonsleeping partner/non-held child family member and non-coworker member of general public	Contribution to sleeping partner from sleeping with patient		TOTAL to co-worker	Contribution to child from patient holding child	
Index Distance (m)				1		
Occupancy Factor	0.25	0.3		0.33	0.3	
		0.33		0.33	0.2	

Time Post-Administration (d)

	If Patient Released at		If Patient Released at		If Patient Released at
Patient releasable if: <**500 mrem (5 mSv)** but must avoid children and pregnant women if >**100 mrem (1 mSv)**	0 d 1 d 2 d		0 d 1 d 2 d		0 d 1 d 2 d 3 d 4 d

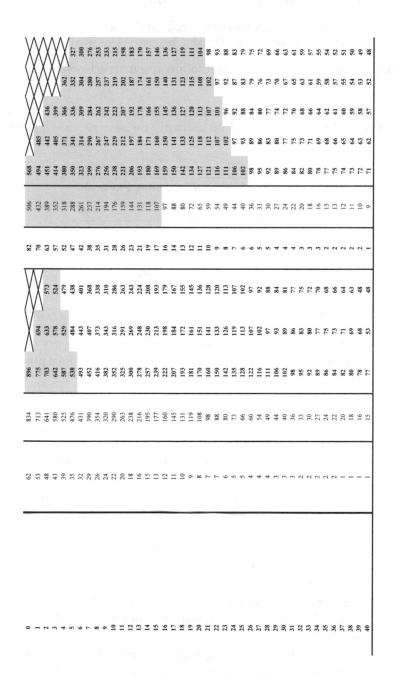

Example 2: Instruction Sheets

Radiation Safety Precautions for Radiopharmaceutical Therapy Patients

Note: Please carefully read and follow the instructions in this document.

If you or your health care provider have any questions or concerns regarding the radionuclide therapy you have received, please contact:

Dr. J. Smith

Nuclear Medicine Attending Physician

at   **(111) 222-3333**

Telephone Number

or   **0000**

Emergency or Pager Telephone Number

Patient **Jane Q. Patient**, Medical Record Number **222-22-222**, received a therapeutic dose of **370 MBq (10 mCi)** of **Iodine-131 Sodium Iodide** at **General Hospital** on **January 1, 2000** at **9:00 am** and *should* observe the following radiation safety precautions at home as follows.

☐ Avoid close contact [less than 1 meter (3 feet) away from] with pregnant women and children until **0 day** after the administration of the radionuclide therapy; that is, there are **no** restrictions on such activity.

☐ However, do not actually hold or embrace children for more than 10 minutes a day until **24 days** after the administration of the radionuclide therapy.

☐ Do not return to work until **0 day** after the administration of the radionuclide therapy; that is, you may return to work **immediately**.

☐ Do not sleep in the same bed with your sleeping partner until **5 days** after the administration of the radionuclide therapy.

☐ However, if your sleeping partner is pregnant, do not sleep in the same bed with your sleeping partner until **29 days** after the administration of the radionuclide therapy.

Patient: **Patient, Jane Q.**
MRN: **222-22-222**

In addition, the following precautions should be observed until 1 day after the administration of your radiopharmaceutical therapy.

- To the extent that is *reasonable*, generally try to remain as far away from individuals around you as possible.
- After using the toilet, flush twice and, as usual, wash your hands. If possible, use paper towels to dry your hands and dispose the paper toweling in the trash.
- You *should* otherwise observe good personal hygiene and may shower, bathe, shave, etc. as you normally would, rinsing the shower stall, tub or sink thoroughly after use.
- Wipe up any spills of urine, saliva and/or mucus with tissues or a small amount of disposable (*i.e.*, flushable) paper toweling, and dispose of the tissue or toweling down the toilet.
- Use nondisposable plates, bowls, spoons, knives, forks and cups. If possible, you *should* wash plates, bowls, spoons, knives, forks and cups which you use, using a separate sponge or wash cloth from that used by the rest of your household. Rinse the sink thoroughly after use, wipe the fixtures with paper towels, and dispose of the paper toweling in the trash.
- If you use a dishwasher, wash your plates, bowls, spoons, knives, forks and cups separately from those of the rest of your household.
- Use the same set of plates, bowls, spoons, knives and forks for 1 day after your radionuclide therapy.
- Store and launder your soiled/used clothing and bed linens separately from those of the rest of your household, running the rinse cycle two times at the completion of machine laundering.
- Do not share food or drinks with anyone.
- After using the telephone, wipe the receiver (especially the mouth piece) with paper towels, and dispose the paper toweling in the trash.

Signature Section (example release form)

I have read this form and all of my questions have been answered. By signing below, I acknowledge that I have read and accept all of the information above.

_____

Signature of patient or personal representative

_____

Print name of patient or personal representative

_____

Date

_____

Relation of personal representative to patient

B.3 Example 3: Metastatic Carcinoid Cancer

In Example 3, a patient with widely metastatic carcinoid cancer was treated with an administered activity of 3.14 GBq (85 mCi) of ^{111}In-DTPA-D-Phe1-Octreotide. Based on kinetic measurements of a pretherapy administration of a 203.5 MBq (5.5 mCi) ^{111}In-DTPA-D-Phe1-Octreotide tracer, this patient was found to exhibit a bi-phasic (bi-exponential) total-body clearance, eliminating 70 and 30 % of the administered activity with effective half-lives of 0.30 and 2.83 d, respectively, yielding an ^{111}In residence time of 1.52 d or 36.6 h. In addition, survey meter measurements immediately following the therapy administration yielded exposure rates of 10 and 113 mR h^{-1} at 1 and 0.3 m, respectively.

Accordingly, because all of the Column 1 values in the spreadsheet are <5 mSv, this patient can be released on the same day of treatment and, because all of these values were actually <1 mSv, the patient need not avoid normal social interactions with children or pregnant women. However, the patient *should* avoid holding small children for >10 min d^{-1} for 18 d after being treated; necessitated by the fact that the values in the "1 d" subcolumn in Column 6 do not decrease to <1 mSv until after day 18 post-treatment. As indicated in the other subcolumns in Column 6, this "child-avoidance" period can be shortened considerably (to as short as 10 d) if the patient avoided children altogether for several days immediately post-treatment.

Because all of the Column 4 values after the first day post-treatment are <1 mSv, the patient can return to work on day two post-treatment. Likewise, subject to the other dose restrictions, general radiation precautions at home are not actually required at all. Nonetheless, it would be prudent to advise the patient to observe such precautions for at least the first day after post-treatment. On the other hand, the patient *should not* sleep in the same bed with a sleeping partner until 5 d after treatment, as the values in the "0 d" subcolumn in Column 3 do not decrease to <5 mSv until day four post-treatment. However, if the patient's sleeping partner is pregnant, her dose limit is lowered to 1 mSv and the patient *should*, therefore, not sleep in the same bed until 21 d after treatment, as the values in the "0 d" subcolumn in Column 3 do not decrease to <1 mSv until after 21 d post-treatment. As indicated in the other subcolumns in Column 3, this period can be shortened considerably if the patient avoided the pregnant sleeping partner altogether for the first several days post-treatment.

The spreadsheet and instructions for this patient are on the following five pages (Zanzonico *et al.*, 2000).

Example 3 Spreadsheet

Times Post-Radionuclide Treatment of Release from Medical Confinement [(t_release)_limit], of Not Working (t_no work), of Avoiding Pregnant Women and Children (t_avoid), of Limited Holding of Children (t_no hold), and of Sleeping Partners Not Sleeping Together (t_sleep apart)

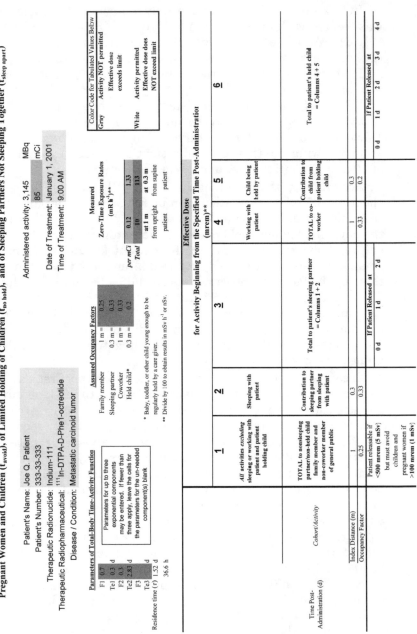

Patient's Name: Joe Q. Patient
Patient's Number: 333-33-333
Therapeutic Radionuclide: Indium-111
Therapeutic Radiopharmaceutical: ¹¹¹In-DTPA-D-Phe1-octreotide
Disease / Condition: Metastatic carcinoid tumor

Administered activity: 3,145   MBq
85   mCi
Date of Treatment: January 1, 2001
Time of Treatment: 9:00 AM

Parameters of Total-Body Time-Activity Function

F1	0.7		Parameters for up to three exponential components may be entered. If fewer than three apply, leave the cells for the parameters for the un-needed component(s) blank
Te1	0.3	d
F2	0.3	
Te2	2.83	d
F3		
Te3		d
Residence time (τ)	1.52	d
	36.6	h

Assumed Occupancy Factors

Family member	1 m =	0.25
Sleeping partner	0.3 m =	0.33
Coworker	1 m =	0.33
Held child*	0.3 m =	0.2

* Baby, toddler, or other child young enough to be regularly held by a care giver.
** Divide by 100 to obtain results in mSv h⁻¹ or nSv.

Measured Zero-Time Exposure Rates (mR h⁻¹)**

per mCi	at 1 m from upright patient	at 0.3 m from supine patient
Total	0.12	1.33
	10	113

Color Code for Tabulated Values Below
Gray: Activity NOT permitted / Effective dose exceeds limit
White: Activity permitted / Effective dose does NOT exceed limit

Effective Dose (mrem)**
for Activity Beginning from the Specified Time Post-Administration

Time Post-Administration (d) — Cohort/Activity	1 — All activities excluding sleeping or working with patient and patient holding child	2 — Sleeping with patient	3 — Total to patient's sleeping partner = Columns 1 + 2	4 — Working with patient	5 — Child being held by patient	6 — Total to patient's held child = Columns 4 + 5
	TOTAL to nonsleeping partner/non-held child family member and non-coworker member of general public	Contribution to sleeping partner from sleeping with patient		Working with patient	Contribution to child from patient holding child	
			If Patient Released at		TOTAL to co-worker	Contribution to child from patient holding child
Index Distance (m)	1	0.3		1	0.3	
Occupancy Factor	0.25	0.33		0.33	0.2	
Patient releasable if <500 mrem (5 mSv) but must avoid children and pregnant women if >100 mrem (1 mSv)			0 d 1 d 2 d			If Patient Released at 0 d 1 d 2 d 3 d 4 d

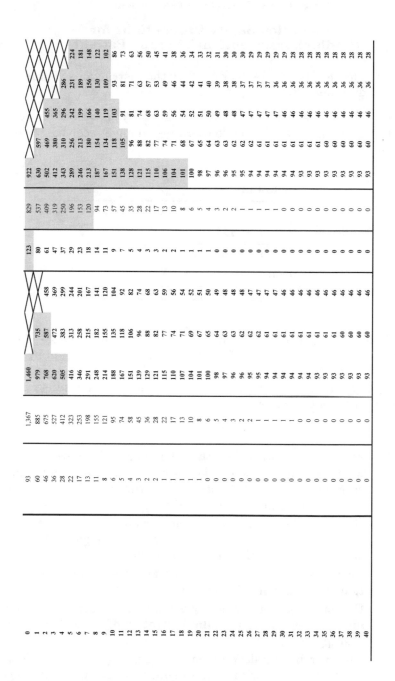

Example 3: Instruction Sheets

Radiation Safety Precautions for Radiopharmaceutical Therapy Patients

Note: Please carefully read and follow the instructions in this document.

If you or your health care provider have any questions or concerns regarding the radionuclide therapy you have received, please contact:

	Dr. J. Smith
	Nuclear Medicine Attending Physician
at	**(111) 222-3333**
	Telephone Number
or	**0000**
	Emergency or Pager Telephone Number

Patient _Joe Q. Patient_, Medical Record Number _333-33-333_, received a therapeutic dose of _3.145 MBq (85 mCi)_ of _Indium-111-DTPA-D-Phel Octreotide_ at _General Hospital_ on _January 1, 2001_ at _9:00 am_ and *should* observe the following radiation safety precautions at home as follows.

☐ Avoid close contact [less than 1 meter (3 feet) away from] with pregnant women and children until _0 days_ after the administration of the radionuclide therapy; that is, there are **no** restrictions on such activity.

☐ However, do not actually hold or embrace children for more than 10 minutes a day until _18 days_ after the administration of the radionuclide therapy.

☐ Do not return to work until _1 day_ after the administration of the radionuclide therapy.

☐ Do not sleep in the same bed with your sleeping partner until _4 days_ after the administration of the radionuclide therapy.

☐ However, if your sleeping partner is pregnant, do not sleep in the same bed with your sleeping partner until _21 days_ after the administration of the radionuclide therapy.

Patient: **Patient, Joe Q.**

MRN: **333-33-333**

In addition, the following precautions should be observed until 1 day after the administration of your radiopharmaceutical therapy.

- To the extent that is *reasonable*, generally try to remain as far away from individuals around you as possible.
- After using the toilet, flush twice and, as usual, wash your hands. If possible, use paper towels to dry your hands and dispose the paper toweling in the trash.
- You *should* otherwise observe good personal hygiene and may shower, bathe, shave, etc. as you normally would, rinsing the shower stall, tub or sink thoroughly after use.
- Wipe up any spills of urine, saliva and/or mucus with tissues or a small amount of disposable (*i.e.*, flushable) paper toweling, and dispose of the tissue or toweling down the toilet.
- Use nondisposable plates, bowls, spoons, knives, forks and cups. If possible, you *should* wash plates, bowls, spoons, knives, forks and cups which you use, using a separate sponge or wash cloth from that used by the rest of your household. Rinse the sink thoroughly after use, wipe the fixtures with paper towels, and dispose of the paper toweling in the trash.
- If you use a dishwasher, wash your plates, bowls, spoons, knives, forks and cups separately from those of the rest of your household.
- Use the same set of plates, bowls, spoons, knives and forks for 1 day after your radionuclide therapy.
- Store and launder your soiled/used clothing and bed linens separately from those of the rest of your household, running the rinse cycle two times at the completion of machine laundering.
- Do not share food or drinks with anyone.
- After using the telephone, wipe the receiver (especially the mouth piece) with paper towels, and dispose the paper toweling in the trash.

Signature Section (example release form)

I have read this form and all of my questions have been answered. By signing below, I acknowledge that I have read and accept all of the information above.

_____

Signature of patient or personal representative

_____

Print name of patient or personal representative

_____

Date

_____

Relation of personal representative to patient

Appendix C

Quality Assurance for High Dose-Rate Brachytherapy Applications

The items presented in this Appendix are intended to provide a template that allows each institution to develop its own QA program. This Appendix cannot be all-inclusive and procedures may differ significantly among the various commercial devices available. As such, these recommendations *should* be viewed as supplemental to QA recommendations from the manufacturers of the various devices. It may also be useful to review the recommendations of other voluntary organizations such as AAPM (Kubo *et al.*, 1998; Kutcher *et al.*, 1994; Nath *et al.*, 1997; Williamson *et al.*, 1994).

Certain QC checks *should* be performed at the start of the treatment day or within 24 h of the start of treatment. Other checks *should* be done immediately before or after treatment.

C.1 Treatment-Preparation Checks

Within 24 h of the start of treatment or at the start of each treatment day, the following items *should* be checked:

- operating condition of reusable applicator systems;
- correct functioning and identity of single-use applicators;
- procedure room preparations;
- correct functioning of remote afterloader;
- operation of treatment-room status indicators and alarm indicator;
- availability of afterloader manual;
- presence and correct functioning of survey instrument;

- functional status of audio/visual communication systems;
- functional status of independent area monitor;
- availability of emergency procedure kit;
- redundant check of assumed source strength;
- spot check of positional accuracy;
- functioning of interlocks at room entrance;
- timer accuracy;
- correct date and time in unit's computer; and
- availability and condition of transfer tubes.

C.2 Applicator Checks

The following items or systems *should* be checked and recorded for each treatment:

- applicator identity *should* be verified and recorded;
- anatomical data needed to identify active dwell positions have been obtained and recorded;
- geometric limitations of the applicator are observed; and
- applicator is correctly assembled.

C.3 Implant Localization and Imaging

Once the applicator has been placed in the patient, imaging of the applicator in the treatment position can be performed. The following data checks *should* be performed:

- applicator(s) is (are) numbered and correctly recorded on the implant diagram;
- multiple applicators, if present, can be distinguished radiographically and correlated with an external numbering system;
- data needed to calculate afterloader-position programming parameters have been measured, recorded and verified;
- imaging parameters (source-film distance, angle, etc.) are correctly recorded; and
- patient name, medical record number, or other identifiers have been recorded on films and in digital systems.

C.4 Treatment Prescription

The treatment prescription *should* be available at the treatment console before and during treatment. The following items *should* be present and reviewed:

- radiation oncologist has signed and reviewed films or images;
- radiation oncologist has signed the treatment prescription;
- radiation oncologist and radiation-oncology physicist have agreed on treatment-planning constraints, dose-specification criteria, and optimization endpoints; and
- radiation oncologist and radiation-oncology physicist have both signed the treatment plan.

C.5 Treatment Planning

The following items *should* be checked before treatment begins:

- programming parameters required by the treatment unit are calculated and independently verified;
- dosimetrist and medical physicist review the planning procedure to be used and agree on reconstruction, optimization and dose-specification procedures to be used;
- dosimetrist or medical physicist verifies patient name on films, prescription and other data, and confirms that the date, time and source strength displayed on planning system. Dosimetrist or medical physicist verifies prescribed dose per fraction against the written prescription; and
- dosimetrist or medical physicist verifies the film orientations, distances, magnifications and gantry angles against requirements for selected reconstruction algorithm.

C.6 Pretreatment Review

This Section is intended to identify the key items to be checked by members of the treatment team. There will be some overlap among these responsibilities, but the responsibility of each person should be clear.

The radiation-oncology physicist *should* review:

- treatment plan and all associated documentation;
- accuracy of critical input data including prescribed dose and source strength;
- positional accuracy;
- accuracy of implant reconstruction;
- independent check of dwell-time calculation accuracy;
- consistency of patient name and identifiers on all documentation; and
- completion of QA measurements.

The radiation oncologist *should* review:

- clinical adequacy of treatment plan and consistency with written prescription;
- target-volume coverage and doses to critical structures; and
- completion of physics checks.

C.7 Patient Setup

The treatment-unit operator, typically a radiation therapist, will place the patient in the treatment position and program treatment parameters verifying the following:

- dose per fraction in treatment plan and prescription agree. The therapist will compare the total dose and number of fractions against treatment(s) previously received;
- agreement between current source strength (*i.e.*, decayed source strength) on treatment plan and the data on the remote afterloader;
- completed prescription is present and signed by both the radiation oncologist and radiation-oncology physicist;
- correct length transfer tubes are being used;
- applicator number and channel number correspond;
- dwell-times and positional settings recorded and displayed by afterloader match the treatment plan;
- identity of patient is verified and matched against the prescription; and
- dose per fraction in the treatment plan is matched against the prescription and the daily treatment record.

C.8 Setup Accuracy

The following additional checks apply to the role of the radiation oncologist and radiation physicist. They *should* ensure that the:

- applicator number and channel number correspond;
- applicator position is checked against measurements made in the operating room and against any reference (fiducial) marks; and
- afterloading programming parameters are verified.

C.9 Treatment

While treatment is in progress, the radiation oncologist (or physician designate), the radiation-oncology physicist, and the radiation-therapist operator *shall* be available during the entire treatment.

C.10 Post-Treatment Checks

At the end of the treatment session and before the patient is released, the following checks *should* be performed:

- patient and personnel safety
  - console indicates source is retracted and treatment is complete;
  - area monitor operation is checked before entering the treatment room and indicates that source is retracted;
  - treatment room is checked with a survey meter to confirm complete retraction of the source(s);
  - HDR device is shut down and secured after the patient is removed; and
  - patient is checked with a survey meter after removal from the treatment room to verify that there are no sources present.
- treatment accuracy and chart order
  - treatment is properly recorded;
  - total dwell-time administered by the device agrees with the calculation; and
  - all forms and checklists are complete and properly filed.

Appendix D

Shielding for High Dose-Rate Brachytherapy Facilities

This Appendix supplements the information presented in Section 5 of this Report. The shielding design approach and the applicable values for shielding design goals (P) recommended for medical-radiation facilities in NCRP Report No. 147 (NCRP, 2004a) and NCRP Report No. 151 (NCRP, 2005) are also recommended for HDR brachytherapy facilities. The reader is referred particularly to NCRP Report No. 147 (NCRP, 2004a) for more detail when the radiation source is limited to low-LET radiation and NCRP Report No. 151 (NCRP, 2005) for considerably more detail on shielding design for other types of radiotherapy facilities, including when high-LET radiation is present.

This Appendix addresses the planning and design of new HDR brachytherapy facilities or the remodeling of existing HDR brachytherapy facilities. HDR brachytherapy facilities designed before the publication of this Report and meeting the requirements of NCRP Report No. 49 (NCRP, 1976) need not be reevaluated (NCRP, 1993b) unless there are changes in a facility's design or use. New equipment, significant changes in the use of existing equipment, or other changes that may have an impact on radiation protection of the staff or members of the public require an evaluation by a qualified expert. This Appendix does not attempt to summarize the regulatory or licensing requirements of the various authorities that may have jurisdiction over matters addressed in this Appendix. It is expected that the qualified expert will be fully aware of these matters and account for them in the final shielding design. While specific recommendations on shielding design methods are

186

presented, alternate methods may prove equally satisfactory in providing adequate radiation protection. The final assessment of the adequacy of the design and construction of protective shielding can only be based on the post-construction radiation survey performed by a qualified expert. If the survey indicates shielding inadequacy, remediation by the addition of shielding or modifications of equipment and procedures *shall* be made. Specific shielding considerations for radiopharmaceutical therapy, other types of brachytherapy, and associated equipment and facilities are discussed throughout Section 5.

The term "qualified expert" as used in this Report and Appendix is defined as a medical physicist or health physicist who is competent to design radiation shielding in radiotherapy facilities, and who is certified by the American Board of Radiology, American Board of Medical Physics, American Board of Health Physics, or Canadian College of Physicists in Medicine. Radiation shielding *shall* be designed by a qualified expert to ensure that the required degree of protection is achieved. The qualified expert *should* be consulted during the early planning stages since the shielding requirements may affect the choice of location and type of building construction. The qualified expert *should* be provided with all pertinent information regarding the proposed radiation equipment and its use, type of building construction, and occupancy of nearby areas. It may also be necessary to submit the final shielding drawings and specifications to pertinent regulatory agencies for review prior to construction.

D.1 General Concepts

The exposure rate from a point radiation source varies inversely as the square of the distance from the source. The exposure time involves both the time that the sealed radioactive source is present outside of a self-shielded housing and the fraction of the treatment time during which a person is present within the radiation field. When the radiation source is brought outside of the shielded housing, sometimes referred to as the "safe," the radiation field will be essentially isotropic. Therefore, the term, use factor (U) (NCRP, 2005), which is typically defined as the fraction of time that a radiation beam is directed toward a shielding barrier, will always be unity for shielding calculations for HDR brachytherapy units. There will be no secondary barriers since all barriers will be exposed to the source as well as to radiation scattered from the patient and objects in the treatment room.

D.1.1 *Occupancy Factor*

The occupancy factor (T) for an area is the average fraction of time that the maximally exposed individual is present while the sealed source is in use and outside of its self-shielded housing. For any particular individual, the occupancy factor is the fraction of the working hours in the week that this individual would occupy the shielded area, averaged over the year. For example, an uncontrolled area adjacent to a treatment room having an assigned occupancy factor of 1/40 would imply that the maximally exposed individual would spend an average of 1 h week^{-1} in that area every workweek for a year.

The occupancy factor for an area is not the fraction of time that it is occupied by any persons, but rather it is the fraction of the time during which it is occupied by the single person who spends the most time there. Thus, a waiting room might be occupied at all times during the working day, but have a very-low occupancy factor since no single person is likely to spend >50 h y^{-1} in any given waiting room. However, if there were to be a receptionist or administrative personnel continuously present in the waiting area, the occupancy factor might approach one.

Occupancy factors in uncontrolled areas will rarely be determined by visitors to the facility or its environs who might be there only for a small fraction of a year. The maximally exposed individual will normally be an employee of the facility. The occupancy factor for controlled areas is usually assigned a value of unity. As mentioned in Section 5 of this Report, Table B.1 of NCRP Report No. 151 (NCRP, 2005) lists suggested occupancy factors for use as a guide in planning shielding.

D.1.2 *Assumptions*

The specified shielding design will be conservatively safe because of the nature of the assumptions made in the shielding design such as:

- attenuation of the radiation within the patient is neglected. The patient typically attenuates the emitted radiation by 30 % or more;
- calculations of recommended barrier thickness often assume perpendicular incidence of the radiation. If the incidence were not perpendicular, the effect would vary in magnitude, but would always result in a reduction in the transmission through the barrier for photons that have nonperpendicular

incidence. This reduction is due to both the increased thickness of the barrier at various angles as well as the resulting increased distance to the barrier;

- minimum distance to the occupied area from a shielded wall is assumed to be 0.3 m. This value is typically a conservatively safe estimate for most walls and especially for doors. If a distance >0.3 m were assumed, the effect would vary, but radiation levels decrease with increasing distance; and
- recommended occupancy factors for uncontrolled areas are typically conservatively high. For example, very few people spend 100 % of their time in their office. If more realistic occupancy factors were to be used, the effect on a calculation would vary in magnitude, but would generally result in a reduction in the amount of exposure received by an individual located in an uncontrolled area.

D.1.3 *Workload*

The units for workload (W) in NCRP Report No. 151 (NCRP, 2005) are Gy week^{-1} at 1 m and conversion to a workload W_n at a distance d_n other than 1 m would be given by $W_n = W \, (1 \text{ m})^2 / (d_n)^2$, a typical inverse square-law calculation. For linear accelerators, the value for W is usually specified as the absorbed dose from photons delivered to the isocenter (*i.e.*, the fixed location around which the machine gantry rotates), in a week, and is selected for each accelerator based on its projected use. A similar concept would apply to HDR brachytherapy units within shielded rooms.

Example: A typical air-kerma rate for an ^{192}Ir HDR unit with a source loading of 370 GBq (10 Ci) would be ~0.039 Gy h^{-1} at 1 m which roughly equates to an absorbed-dose rate of 0.043 Gy h^{-1} at 1 m. This information and the number of patients treated per day, treatment time per patient, and number of treatment days per week of operation are used to determine the workload.

For a treatment load of four patients per day with an average treatment time of 20 min per patient, the treatment time per day would be 80 min. Assuming a treatment schedule of 5 d week^{-1}, the total treatment time per week would be 400 min or ~6.7 h week^{-1}. Multiplying this value by the absorbed-dose rate at 1 m, 0.043 Gy h^{-1}, yields a workload of 0.3 Gy week^{-1}.

Workload estimates *should* also include an estimate of the absorbed dose delivered during QC checks, calibrations, or other physics measurements. If the calibration, QC checks, or other physics measurements are made at distances or locations other than the treatment distance and location, a separate assessment *should* be made for the distance and occupancy factors that may apply.

If the HDR unit were to be located within another treatment room (*e.g.*, a linear accelerator room) that is also used for patient treatment, the number of treatment hours available for HDR treatments may be limited by the schedule for the other treatment modalities. The required shielding for the treatment room will be determined by the total workload for all the radiotherapy equipment located in the room.

D.1.4 *Location of the Treatment*

The location of the treatment table or couch within the treatment room will be used to determine the distance from the source to the shielded area. There are a number of potential locations for a treatment couch, including the following:

- when the HDR unit is located within a treatment room designated for other types of radiation treatments (*e.g.*, an HDR unit within a linear accelerator vault) the accelerator treatment table within the room may serve as the HDR treatment couch. Typically, this requires adding devices to the treatment couch (*e.g.*, stirrups) so that the patient can be positioned for treatment;

- when the HDR unit is located within a treatment room as above, a separate treatment table may be stored with the HDR unit. This table would only be used for HDR treatments. When in use, the treatment table would need to be positioned within the field of view of cameras located within the treatment room. Typically, at least two cameras are present within the treatment room, one near-field and one far-field camera, which allow the patient to be viewed during treatment; and

- a separate facility may be available for HDR treatment and this facility may use a standard examining table equipped for urological or gynecological treatment.

In any of the examples noted above, the distance from the source to the shielded area may vary. However, it is important to define clearly the limits of positioning and the distances to the areas to be protected.

D.1.5 *Source Parameter*

Currently available commercial HDR units use sources of ^{192}Ir with activities varying between 370 GBq (10 Ci) and 444 GBq (12 Ci). Several manufacturers are hoping to increase the available sealed source activity to 555 GBq (15 Ci). Various authors have explored the use of [169]Yb for brachytherapy and more recently the use of [170]Tm has also been proposed (Das *et al.*, 1997; Granero *et al.*, 2006; Williamson, 1996). These radionuclides combine the possibility of high specific activity with the emission of low-energy photons. As compared to ^{192}Ir, the shielding for the lower energy radionuclides will be reduced in thickness. Table D.1 lists the half-value layers (HVL) and tenth-value layers (TVL) for ^{192}Ir and [169]Yb. The first TVL and equilibrium tenth-value layers (TVL$_e$) values are used to account for the changes in the radiation spectrum that occur as the radiation penetrates the barrier. For the values given in Table D.1, lead density was taken to be 11.36 g cm^{-3} and concrete density was taken to be 2.3 g cm^{-3}.

Two literature references have recently presented the results of Monte-Carlo simulations for various parameters used in shielding for HDR units (Granero *et al.*, 2006; Lymperopoulou *et al.*, 2006). Figures D.1 and D.2 present transmission curves in lead and concrete for three HDR sealed sources, one that is in use currently and the other two that have the potential for future use in HDR brachytherapy.

D.2 Construction Inspection

It is recommended that a qualified expert carry out physical inspections of the facility during construction. The inspections *should* include, at a minimum, an evaluation of the following items:

- thickness and density of concrete, if used;
- thickness of lead shielding, if used;
- heating, ventilation and air conditioning, and shielding baffles, as necessary;
- location and size of conduit(s) or pipe used for electrical cables, including cables for control consoles and machine operation, plumbing or other penetrations of the shielding; and
- verification that the shielding design has been followed.

It is often impractical to make an overall experimental determination of the adequacy of the shielding prior to the completion of

TABLE D.1—*Values for lead and concrete for HVL, HVL$_e$, TVL, and TVL$_e$ for ^{192}Ir and ^{169}Yb (Lymperopoulou, 2006).*

	First HVL	HVL$_e$	First TVL	TVL$_e$
	Lead thickness (mm)			
^{192}Ir	2.8	5.7	11.0	18.7
	3[a]	6[b]	12[a]	20[b]
^{169}Yb	0.25	1.6	1.8	5.3
	0.23[c]	—	2[a]	—
	Concrete thickness (cm)			
^{192}Ir	6.5	4.2	17.6	14.1
	—	3[b]	—	4.7[b]
	3.2	3.4	10.6	11.4
	2.7[c]	—	10.4[c]	—

[a]Values reported in Lymperopoulou *et al.* (2006) and taken from Delacroix (1998).
[b]Values reported in Lymperopoulou *et al.* (2006) and taken from NCRP (1976).
[c]Values reported in Lymperopoulou *et al.* (2006) and taken from Granero (2006). Lead density was taken to be 11.36 g cm^{-3} and concrete density was taken to be 2.3 g cm^{-3}.

the building construction and the installation of the radiotherapy equipment. Periodic inspections during the entire construction period *should* be performed. Sometimes properly constructed shielding is compromised by subsequent changes that are made to install ducts, recessed boxes, or other hardware. These alterations can be made to walls, ceilings or floors. Hence, there *should* be periodic checks of the continued validity of shielding assumptions and the integrity of the barriers.

The shielding of the treatment room *shall* be constructed so that the shielding is not compromised by joints, by openings for ducts, pipes or other objects passing through the barriers, or by conduits, service boxes, or other structural elements embedded in the shielding barriers. Other aspects of facility design, such as interlocks, warning signs, warning lights, electrical safety, and room lighting are discussed briefly in NCRP Report No. 151 and are discussed in more detail in NCRP Report No. 102 (NCRP, 1989; 2005). A

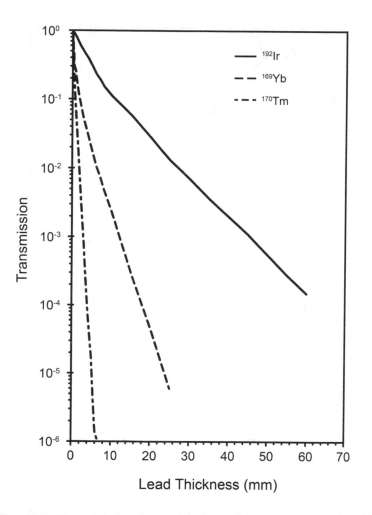

Fig. D.1. Transmission as a function of lead thickness for ^{192}Ir, ^{169}Yb, and ^{170}Tm (lead density is taken as 11.36 g cm^{-3}).

summary document outlining the results of the construction inspection *shall* be prepared by the qualified expert and forwarded, as appropriate, to the owner of the facility, the architectural firm involved in the construction and any governing regulatory agency, as necessary. Any items of noncompliance *shall* be clearly indicated and recommendations for remediation *should* be made.

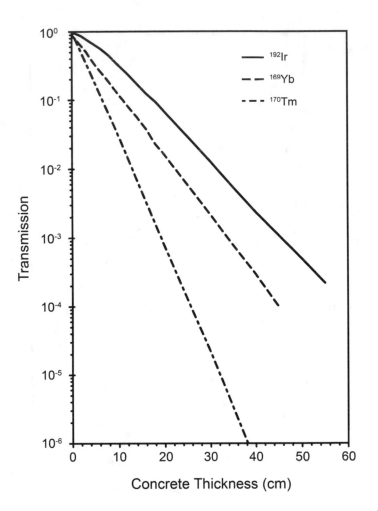

Fig. D.2. Transmission as a function of concrete thickness for ^{192}Ir, ^{169}Yb, and ^{170}Tm (concrete density is taken as 2.35 g cm^{-3}).

D.3 Performance Assessment

After construction, a performance assessment (*i.e.*, a radiation survey), including measurements in controlled and uncontrolled areas, *shall* be made by a qualified expert to confirm that the shielding provided will achieve the applicable shielding design goals for controlled and uncontrolled areas. This performance assessment is an independent check that the assumptions used in the shielding design are conservatively safe. For a discussion of shielding evaluations [see Section 6.4 of NCRP Report No. 151 (NCRP, 2005)].

D.4 Documentation Requirements

The following documentation *shall* be maintained on a permanent basis by the owner of the facility:

- shielding design report, including assumptions and specifications;
- construction, or preferably as-built, documents showing location and amounts of shielding material installed;
- post-construction survey reports;
- information regarding remediation, if any were required; and
- any subsequent evaluations of the room shielding relative to changes (*e.g.*, in utilization) that have been made or are under consideration.

Glossary

absorbed dose (*D*): Quotient of $d\bar{\varepsilon}$ by dm, where $d\bar{\varepsilon}$ is the mean energy imparted by ionizing radiation to matter in a volume element and dm is the mass of matter in that volume element: $D = d\bar{\varepsilon}/dm$. For purposes of radiation protection and assessing dose or risk to humans in general terms, the quantity normally calculated is the mean absorbed dose in an organ or tissue (T): $D_T = \bar{\varepsilon}_T/m_T$, where $\bar{\varepsilon}$ is the total energy imparted in an organ or tissue of mass m_T. The SI unit of absorbed dose is the joule per kilogram (J kg^{-1}), and its special name is the gray (Gy). In conventional units often used by federal and state agencies, absorbed dose is given in rad; 1 rad = 0.01 Gy.

activity (*A*): Rate of transformation (disintegration or decay) of radioactive material. The SI unit of activity is the reciprocal second (s^{-1}), and its special name is the becquerel (Bq). In conventional units often used by federal and state agencies, activity is given in curies (Ci); 1 Ci = 3.7×10^{10} Bq.

administered activity (*AA*): The amount, in terms of activity, of radioactive source material given to a patient during a diagnostic or therapeutic procedure. (Although the term "dose" is often used in practice in referring to the administered activity, the latter quantity is not the same as absorbed dose.)

air kerma (kerma) (kinetic energy released per unit of mass) (*K*): The quotient of the sum of the initial kinetic energies of all the charged particles liberated by uncharged particles in matter divided by the mass of the matter into which the particles are released and is given the special name gray (Gy). 1 Gy = 1 J kg^{-1}. In the event that the matter is air, kerma is often referred to as air kerma.

air-kerma strength (S_K): Product of the air-kerma rate and the square of the distance. The units of air-kerma strength are µGy m^2 h^{-1} or cGy cm^2 h^{-1}.

as low as reasonably achievable (ALARA): Principle of radiation protection that calls for every reasonable effort to maintain radiation exposures as far below specified limits as is practical, taking into account cost-benefit and any other societal concerns.

becquerel (Bq): SI special name for the unit of activity. 1 Bq equals one disintegration per second. 37 MBq (megabecquerels) = 1 mCi (millicurie) (see **curie**).

brachytherapy: Method of radiation therapy in which an encapsulated source is utilized to deliver gamma or beta radiation at a distance up to a few centimeters either by surface, intracavitary or interstitial application.

chart: A patient's medical record or treatment folder in written or electronic (computerized) format that is the permanent institutional document in a medical facility and that fully describes the medical history and care of the patient.

contamination: Radioactive material suspended in air or deposited in any area or on any surface where its presence is unwanted or unexpected.

controlled area: Limited-access area in which the occupational exposure of personnel to radiation is under the supervision of an individual in charge of radiation protection. This definition implies that access, occupancy and working conditions are controlled for purposes of radiation protection.

curie (Ci): Conventional special name for the unit of activity equal to 3.70×10^{10} becquerels (or disintegrations per second) (see **becquerel**).

deterministic effects: Detrimental health effects for which the severity varies with the dose of radiation (or other toxic substance), and for which a threshold usually exists.

dose equivalent (H): Absorbed dose (D) at a point in tissue weighted by quality factor (Q) for type and energy of the radiation causing the dose: $H = D \times Q$. For purposes of radiation protection and assessing health risks in general terms, and especially prior to introduction of the equivalent dose and as used by federal and state agencies, dose equivalent often refers to mean absorbed dose in an organ or tissue (T) weighted by average quality factor ($\overline{Q}$) for the particular type of radiation: $H_T = D_T \times \overline{Q}$. The SI unit of dose equivalent is the joule per kilogram (J kg^{-1}), and its special name is the sievert (Sv). In conventional units often used by federal and state agencies, dose equivalent is given in rem; 1 rem = 0.01 Sv

dose limit (E_{limit}): Limit on effective dose that is applied for exposure to individuals in order to prevent the occurrence of radiation induced deterministic effects and to limit the probability of radiation-related stochastic effects to an acceptable level.

effective dose (E): Sum over specified organs and tissues (T) of mean **dose equivalent** in each tissue weighted by **tissue weighting factor** (w_T):. It is given by the expression:

$$E = \sum w_T H_T, \tag{G.1}$$

where H_T is the equivalent dose in tissue or organ T and w_T is the tissue weighting factor for tissue or organ T. The unit for E and H_T is joule per kilogram (J kg^{-1}) with the special name of sievert (Sv). 1 Sv = 1 J kg^{-1} (supersedes **effective dose equivalent**).

equivalent dose (H_T): Mean absorbed dose in a tissue or organ weighted by the radiation weighting factor (w_R) for the type and energy of radiation incident on the body. The equivalent dose in tissue or organ T is given by the expression:

$$H_T = \sum w_R D_{T,R},$$
(G.2)

where $D_{T,R}$ is the mean absorbed dose in the tissue or organ T due to radiation type R. The SI unit of equivalent dose is the joule per kilogram (J kg^{-1}) with the special name sievert (Sv). 1 Sv = 1 J kg^{-1}.

exposure (X): Most often used in a general sense meaning to be irradiated. When used as the specifically defined radiation quantity, exposure is a measure of the ionization produced in air by x or gamma radiation. The unit of exposure is coulomb per kilogram (C kg^{-1}). The special unit for exposure is roentgen (R), where 1 R = 2.58 × 10^{-4} C kg^{-1}.

family member: Any person who provides support and comfort to a patient on a regular basis and is considered by the patient as a member of their "family" whether by birth or marriage or by virtue of a close, loving relationship.

gray (Gy): SI special name for the unit of the quantities absorbed dose and air kerma. 1 Gy = 1 J kg^{-1}.

half-life ($T_{1/2}$): Time required to reduce spontaneously the activity of a radionuclide to one-half of the activity originally present. Physical or radioactive half-life refers to reduction of activity by radioactive decay; biological half-life refers to elimination of the activity by biological processes; and effective half-life refers to the combined action of radioactive decay and biological elimination.

high dose rate (HDR): As used in brachytherapy, HDR refers to a type of remote afterloader housed in a treatment room that contains a high activity source of radiation used to deliver a therapeutic treatment to a patient in a relatively short treatment time.

implant: A completed assembly of radioactive sealed sources with or without applicators that is placed in a patient with therapeutic intent.

integrated reference air kerma (*IRAK*): Special term used in brachytherapy for integrated reference air kerma strength, a product of S_K and treatment time. The unit of *IRAK* is Gy m^2.

kerma (K): (see **air kerma**).

low dose rate (LDR): As used in brachytherapy, LDR refers to the use of sealed sources placed in a patient on a permanent or temporary basis to deliver a therapeutic dose of radiation.

medical facility: A hospital, clinic or other facility that may practice radiation therapy with sealed sources or radiopharmaceuticals and that provides in-patient care. This definition specifically excludes the patient's own home.

medical health physicist: (see **qualified expert**).

medical physicist (medical-radiation physicist): (see **qualified expert**).

member of the public: In the context of possible radiation exposure from a radioactive patient, this term refers to any individual, not a member of the patient's family and not an individual exposed to radiation in the course of their employment.

milligrams radium equivalent (mgRaEq): Strength of a given source in milligrams radium equivalent is the mass in milligram of ^{226}Ra, encapsulated in a cylinder with wall thickness of 0.5 mm platinum-iridium, that gives the same transverse-axis radiation output, or air-kerma strength, as the source itself.

nuclear-medicine physician: Physician licensed to practice medicine who is qualified by training and experience to be authorized under the facility's license to prescribe the administration of therapeutic amounts of radiopharmaceuticals. Use of the term "nuclear-medicine physician" does not require that the physician be part of a facility's nuclear-medicine group.

occupational exposures: Radiation exposures to individuals that are incurred in the workplace as a result of situations that can reasonably be regarded as being the responsibility of management (exposures associated with medical diagnosis of or treatment for the individual are excluded).

preloaded applications: "Hot source" brachytherapy technique that consists of placing the radioactive sources manually or placing applicators previously loaded with radioactive sources in the treatment site during an operative procedure.

qualified expert: A medical physicist or medical health physicist, who is competent to design radiation shielding, evaluate the results of radiation dosimetry measurements, and specify radiation precautions to be observed when administering or handling radioactive materials. The qualified expert is a physicist certified by the American Board of Radiology, American Board of Medical Physics, American Board of Health Physics, or the Canadian College of Physicists in Medicine.

rad: Special name for the conventional unit of absorbed dose. 1 rad = 0.01 J kg^{-1}. In the SI system of units, it is replaced by the special name gray (Gy). 1 Gy = 100 rad.

radiation oncologist: Physician licensed to practice medicine who is qualified by training and experience to prescribe the administration of brachytherapy treatment. Use of the term "radiation oncologist" does not require that this physician be part of a facility's radiation-oncology department or group. In certain jurisdictions, the qualifications required under the appropriate regulatory authority may also be met by osteopaths.

radiation safety officer (RSO): An individual who meets the applicable regulatory requirements of training and experience to be named on a facility's license as the RSO. Depending on the license and complexity of the program, the RSO may be a nuclear-medicine physician, a radiologist, a radiation oncologist, a nuclear pharmacist, a medical physicist, or a medical health physicist. Facilities may use alternate titles such as radiation protection supervisor or radiation safety manager. Throughout this Report, any reference to the RSO is intended to include individuals designated by the RSO such as radiation safety staff.

radiation weighting factor (w_R): Dimensionless weighting factor developed for purposes of radiation protection and assessing health risks in general terms that accounts for relative biological effectiveness of different types (and, in some cases, energies) of radiations in producing **stochastic effects** and is used to relate mean **absorbed dose** in an organ or tissue (T) to **equivalent dose**. The radiation weighting factor is intended to supersede the mean quality factor ($\overline{Q}$) and is defined with respect to the type and energy of the radiation incident on the body or, in the case of sources within the body, emitted by the source. Radiation weighting factor is independent of **tissue weighting factor** (w_T).

radiopharmaceutical: Radioactive substance administered to a patient for diagnostic or therapeutic nuclear-medicine procedures. A radiopharmaceutical contains two parts, the radionuclide and the pharmaceutical (*e.g.*, ^{99m}Tc DTPA). In some cases the two are one (*e.g.*, ^{133}Xe gas).

rem: Special name for the conventional unit numerically equal to the absorbed dose (D) in rad, modified by a quality factor (Q). 1 rem = 0.01 J kg^{-1}. In the SI system of units, it is replaced by the special name sievert (Sv), which is numerically equal to the absorbed dose (D) in gray modified by a radiation weighting factor (w_R). 1 Sv = 100 rem.

roentgen (R): Special name for the unit of exposure. Exposure is a specific quantity of ionization (charge) produced by the absorption of x- or gamma-radiation energy in a specified mass of air under standard conditions. 1 R = 2.58×10^{-4} coulomb per kilogram (C kg^{-1}).

sievert (Sv): Special name for the SI unit of dose equivalent, equivalent dose, and effective dose. 1 Sv = 1 J kg^{-1}.

specific bremsstrahlung constant (Γ_{br}): Constant that relates the activity in a point source of beta-emitting radiation to the bremsstrahlung exposure rate from that source. The unit of the specific bremsstrahlung constant is R cm^2 mCi^{-1} h^{-1}.

specific gamma-ray constant (Γ_γ): Constant that relates the activity in a point source of penetrating radiation (photons) to the exposure rate from the source. The units of the specific gamma-ray constant is R cm^2 mCi^{-1} h^{-1}, equivalent to the exposure rate in air in R h^{-1} at 1 cm from a 1 mCi source. The specific gamma-ray constant is unique to the radionuclide under consideration.

stochastic effects: Adverse effects in biological organisms for which the probability, but not the severity, is assumed to be a function of dose of ionizing radiation (or other contaminant) without threshold.

survey meter: Instrument or device, usually portable, for monitoring the level of radiation or of radioactive contamination in an area or location.

tissue weighting factor (w_T): Dimensionless factor that represents ratio of the stochastic risk attributable to a specific organ or tissue (T) to total stochastic risk attributable to all organs and tissues when the whole body receives a uniform exposure to ionizing radiation. When calculating effective dose equivalent, tissue weighting factor represents the risk of fatal cancers or severe hereditary effects. When calculating effective dose, tissue weighting factor represents total detriment.

treatment folder: (see **chart**).

use factor (*U*) (beam direction factor): Fraction of the workload during which the useful beam is directed at the barrier under consideration.

Symbols and Acronyms

A	activity
$\tilde{A}$	cumulated activity in a patient per unit administered activity AA
AA	activity administered to a patient
ALARA	as low as reasonably achievable
$A(t)$	total body activity at post-administration time
CT	computed tomography
d	distance
D	absorbed dose
$\dot{D}_r$	absorbed-dose rate in a medium at distance r
DTPA	diethelyene triamine pentaacetic acid
$D_{T,R}$	mean absorbed dose for tissue T and radiation type R
E	effective dose, summation of all $H_T \times w_T$
$E\,K_a^{-1}$	effective dose per unit air-kerma conversion coefficient
E_{limit}	effective dose limits for radiation protection
E_p	photon energy
$\dot{E}(r_j,t)$	effective dose rate at a distance at a post-administration time
$E(r_j)_{t_1 \to t_2}$	effective dose at a distance at a post-administration time period
ERT	external-beam radiotherapy
F_i	zero time intercept of total body activity of exponential component i
GM	Geiger-Muller
H	dose equivalent
HDR	high dose rate
$H_p(d)$	personal dose equivalent at a depth in tissue
H_T	equivalent dose to tissue organ, the summation of all $H_{T,R}$
$H_{T,R}$	equivalent dose, $D_{T,R} \times w_R$
HVL	half-value layer
HVL_e	equilibrium half-value layer

IRAK	integrated reference air kerma
ISO	isotropic
K_a	air kerma
$(K_{a_b})^{med}_{air}$	ratio of the air kerma in the medium to that in air at distance r from the source
$\dot{K}_a(r_j,t)$	air kerma rate at a distance at a post-administration time
LDR	low dose rate
LET	linear energy transfer
MCPT	Monte-Carlo photon transport
μ	linear attenuation coefficient
$\left(\dfrac{\mu_{en}}{\rho}\right)^{med}_{air}$	mass-energy absorption coefficient ratio to convert air kerma to absorbed dose in a medium
n	number of exponential components required to describe time-dependent total-body activity
P	shielding design goal
PET	positron-emission tomography
PET/CT	positron-emission tomography combined with computed tomography
PDR	pulsed dose rate
PTA	percutaneous transluminal balloon angioplasty
PTCA	percutaneous transluminal coronary angioplasty
Q	quality factor
QA	quality assurance
QC	quality control
r	distance from the radioactive source
ρ	density
ROT	rotational
RSC	radiation safety committee
RSO	radiation safety officer
S_K	air-kerma strength
T	occupancy factor
τ	residence time of activity in patient
T_e	effective half-life of the nondecay corrected total-body activity for a single exponential function
T_{e_i}	effective half-life of the nondecay corrected total-body activity for component i of a multi-exponential function

t_{avoid}	period for avoiding women and children
$t_{no\ hold}$	period for not holding children
$t_{no\ work}$	period for not working after release from medical confinement
$t_{sleep\ apart}$	period for sleeping partners not sleeping together
T_p	physical half-life
Γ_{br}	specific bremsstrahlung constant (Table 3.1)
Γ_γ	specific gamma-ray constant
Γ_δ	exposure-rate constant
$(t_{release})_{limit}$	time of patient release from medical confinement based on particular effective-dose limit
T_{r_j}	occupancy factor for an individual at a distance from a radioactive patient
TVL	tenth-value layer
TVL_e	equilibrium tenth-value layer
U	unit of air-kerma strength
U	use factor
W	workload
w_R	radiation weighting factor
w_T	tissue weighting factor
X	exposure

References

ABRAMSON, D.H., FASS, D., MCCORMICK, B., SERVODIDIO, C.A., PIRO, J.D. and ANDERSON, L.L. (1997). "Implant brachytherapy: A novel treatment for recurrent orbital rhabdomyosarcoma," J. Am. Assoc. Pediat. Ophthalmol. Strabismus 1(3), 154 – 157.

AMOLS, H.I. (2002). "Intravascular brachytherapy physics: Review of radiation sources and techniques," pages 223 to 240 in *Vascular Brachytherapy*, 3rd. ed., Waksman, R.E., Ed. (Futura Publishing Company, Armonk, New York).

AMOLS, H.I., ZAIDER, M., WEINBERGER, J., ENNIS, R., SCHIFF, P. and REINSTEIN, L. (1996a). "Dosimetric considerations for catheter-based beta and gamma emitters in the therapy of neointimal hyperplasia in human coronary arteries," Int. J. Radiat. Oncol. Biol. Phys. 36(4), 913–921.

AMOLS, H.I., REINSTEIN, L.E. and WEINBERGER, J. (1996b). "Dosimetry of a radioactive coronary balloon dilation catheter for treatment of neointimal hyperplasia," Med. Phys. 23(10), 1783–1788.

ANDERSON, L.L., NATH, R., WEAVER, K.A., NORI, D., PHILLIPS, T.L., SON, Y.H., CHIU-TSAO, S.T., MEIGOONI, A.S., MELI, J.A. and SMITH, V. (1990). *Interstitial Brachytherapy, Physical, Biological, and Clinical Considerations* (Raven Press, New York).

ANDERSON, L.L., MONI, J.V. and HARRISON, L.B. (1993). "A nomograph for permanent implants of ^{103}Pd seeds," Int. J. Radiat. Oncol. Biol. Phys. 27(1), 129–135.

ANDERSON, L.L., HARRINGTON, P.J. and ST. GERMAIN, J. (1999). "Physics of intraoperative high dose rate brachytherapy," pages 87 to 104 in *Intraoperative Irradiation, Techniques and Results*, Gunderson, L., Willet, C., Harrison, L. and Calvo, F., Eds. (Humana Press, Totowa, New Jersey).

ANSI (1996). American National Standards Institute. *Performance Criteria for Radiobioassay*, BSR N13.30 (American National Standards Institute, New York).

ANSI (2001). American National Standards Institute. *Performance and Documentation of Radiation Surveys*, ANSI N13.49 (American National Standards Institute, New York).

BAKHEET, S.M., POWE, J. and HAMMAMI, M.M. (1998). "Unilateral radioiodine breast uptake," Clin. Nucl. Med. 23(3), 170–171.

BALACHANDRAN, S., MCGUIRE, L., FLANIGAN, S., SHAH, H. and BOYD, C.M. (1985). "Bremsstrahlung imaging after ^{32}P treatment for residual suprasellar cyst," Int. J. Nucl. Med. Biol. 12(3), 215–221.

BALTER, S., OETGEN, M., HILL, A., DALTON, J., SACHER, A., LIPSZTEIN, R., COLLINS, M. and MOSES, J. (2000). "Personnel exposure during gamma endovascular brachytherapy," Health Phys. **79**(2), 136–146.

BANDER, N.H., NANUS, D.M., MILOWSKY, M.I., KOSTAKOGLU, L., VALLABAHAJOSULA, S. and GOLDSMITH, S.J. (2003). "Targeted systemic therapy of prostate cancer with a monoclonal antibody to prostate-specific membrane antigen," Semin. Oncol. **30**(5), 667–676.

BARRINGTON, S.F., KETTLE, A.G., O'DOHERTY, M.J., WELLS, C.P., SOMER, E.J. and COAKLEY, A.J. (1996). "Radiation dose rates from patients receiving ^{131}I therapy for carcinoma of the thyroid," Eur. J. Nucl. Med. **23**(2), 123–130.

BARRINGTON, S.F., O'DOHERTY, M.J., KETTLE, A.G., THOMSON, W.H., MOUNTFORD, P.J., BURRELL, D.N., FARRELL, R.J., BATCHELOR, S., SEED, P. and HARDING, L.K. (1999). "Radiation exposure of the families of outpatients treated with radioiodine (^{131}I) for hyperthyroidism," Eur. J. Nucl. Med. **26**(7), 686–692.

BENUA, R.S., CICALE, N.R., SONENBERG, M. and RAWSON, R.W. (1962). "The relation of radioiodine dosimetry to results and complications in the treatment of metastatic thyroid cancer," Am. J. Roentgenol. Ther. Nucl. Med. **87**, 171–182.

BLAKE, G.M., ZIVANOVIC, M.A., BLAQUIERE, R.M., FINE, D.R., MCEWAN, A.J. and ACKERY, D.M. (1988). "Strontium-89 therapy: Measurement of absorbed dose to skeletal metastases," J. Nucl. Med. **29**(4), 549–557.

BLASKO, J.C., RAGDE, H. and SCHUMACKER, D. (1987). "Transperineal percutaneous ^{125}I implantation for prostatic carcinoma using transrectal ultrasound and template guidance," Endocuriether. Hyperther. Oncol. **3**, 131–139.

BOHAN, M., YUE, N. and NATH, R. (2000). "On the need for massive additional shielding of a catheterization laboratory for the implementation of high dose rate ^{192}Ir intravascular brachytherapy," Cardiovasc. Radiat. Med. **2**, 39–4.

BOYE, E., LINDEGAARD, M.W., PAUS, E., SKRETTING, A., DAVY, M. and JAKOBSEN, E. (1984). "Whole-body distribution of radioactivity after intraperitoneal administration of ^{32}P colloids," Br. J. Radiol. **57**(677), 395–402.

BREEN, S.L., POWE, J.E. and PORTER, A.T. (1992). "Dose estimation in strontium-89 radiotherapy of metastatic prostatic carcinoma," J. Nucl. Med. **33**(7), 1316–1323.

BRUCER, M. (1993). "William Duane and the radium cow: An American contribution to an emerging atomic age," Med. Phys. **20**(6), 1601–1605.

BUCHANAN, R.C. and BRINDLE, J.M. (1970). "Radioiodine therapy to out-patients: The contamination hazard," Br. J. Radiol. **43**, 479–482.

BUCHANAN, R. and BRINDLE, J. (1971) "Radioiodine therapy to out-patients: The radiation hazard," Br. J. Radiol. **44**, 973–975.

BUYS, R.J., ABRAMSON, D.H., ELLSWORTH, R.M. and HAIK, B. (1983). "Radiation regression patterns after cobalt plaque insertion for retinoblastoma," Arch. Opthalmol. **101**(8), 1206–1208.

CALLAN, J.R., KELLY, R.T., QUINN, M.L., GWYNNE, J.W. MOORE, R.A., MUCKLER, F.A., KASUMOVIC, J., SAUNDERS, W.M., LEPAGE, R.P., CHIN, E., SCHOENFELD, I. and SERIG, D.I. (1995). *Human Factors Evaluation of Remote Afterloading Brachytherapy: Human Error and Critical Tasks in Remote Afterloading Brachytherapy and Approaches for Improved System Performance*, NUREG/CR-6125, Vol. 1 (U.S. Nuclear Regulatory Commission, Washington).

CAMPBELL, A.M., BAILEY, I.H. and BURTON, M.A. (2000). "Analysis of the distribution of intra-arterial microspheres in human liver following hepatic ^{90}Y microsphere therapy," Phys. Med. Biol. **45**(4), 1023–1033.

CASARA, D., RUBELLO, D., SALADINI, G., PIOTTO, A., PELIZZO, M.R., GIRELLI, M.E. and BUSNARDO, B. (1993). "Pregnancy after high therapeutic doses of ^{131}I in differentiated thyroid cancer: Potential risks and recommendations," Eur. J. Nucl. Med. **20**(3), 192–194.

CHENERY, S.G., PLA, M. and PODGORSAK, E.B. (1985). "Physical characteristics of the selectron high dose rate intracavitary afterloader," Br. J. Radiol. **58**(692), 735–740.

CHEUNG, N.K., KUSHNER, B.H. and KRAMER, K. (2001). "Monoclonal antibody-based therapy of neuroblastoma," Hematol. Oncol. Clin. North Am. **15**(5), 853–866.

CODY, H.S., III, Ed. (2002). *Sentinel Lymph Node Biopsy* (Martin Dinitz Publishers, Ltd., London).

COOLIDGE, W.D. (1913). "A powerful roentgen ray tube with a pure electron discharge," Phys. Rev. **2**(6), 409–430.

CONTI, P.S., WHITE, C., PIESLOR, P., MOLINA, A., AUSSIE, J. and FOSTER, P. (2005). "The role of imaging with ^{111}In-ibritumomab tiuxetan in the ibritumomab tiuxetan (Zevalin®) regimen: Results from a Zevalin® imaging registry," J. Nucl. Med. **46**(11), 1812–1818.

CORMACK, J. and SHEARER, J. (1998). "Calculation of radiation exposures from patients to whom radioactive materials have been administered," Phys. Med. Biol. **43**(3), 501–516.

CULVER, C.M. and DWORKIN, H.J. (1991). "Radiation safety considerations for post-^{131}I hyperthyroid cancer therapy," J. Nucl. Med. **32**(1), 169–173.

CULVER, C.M. and DWORKIN, H.J. (1992). "Radiation safety considerations for post-^{131}I thyroid cancer therapy," J. Nucl. Med. **33**(7), 1402–1405.

CURIE, E. (1938). *Madame Curie, A Biography* (Doubleday-Doran, New York).

CURIE, P., CURIE, M. and BELMONT, G. (1898). "Sur une nouvelle substance fortement radioactive contenue dans la petchblende," Comptes Rendus. Acad. Sci. Paris **127**, 1215–1217.

DAM, H.J.W. (1896). "The new marvel in photography. A visit to Professor Roentgen at his laboratory in Wurzburg – his own account of his great discovery – interesting experiments with the cathode rays. Practical uses of the new photography," http://www.ibiblio.org/pub/docs/books/

gutenberg/1/4/6/6/14663/14663-8.txt (accessed May 24, 2007) McClure's Mag. **6**(5).

DAS, R.K., MEIGOONI, A.S., MISHRA, V., LANGTON, M.A. and WILLIAMSON, J.F. (1997). "Dosimetric characteristics of the type 8 ^{169}Yb interstitial brachytherapy source," J. Brachyther. Int. **13**, 219–234.

DAUER, L.T., ZELEFSKY, M.J, HORAN, C., YAMADA, Y. and ST. GERMAIN, J. (2004). "Assessment of radiation safety instructions to patients based on measured dose rates following prostate brachytherapy," Brachytherapy **3**(1), 1–6.

DEGUZMAN, A.F., KEARNS, W.T., SHAW, F., TATTER, S., STIEBER, V., YATES, C., AMADEO, H. and HINSON, W.H. (2003). "Radiation safety issues with high activities of liquid ^{125}I: Techniques and experience," J. Appl. Clin. Med. Phys. **4**(2), 143–148.

DEHEVESY, G. (1948). *Radioactive Indicators; Their Application in Biochemistry, Animal Physiology and Pathology* (Interscience Publishers, New York).

DELACROIX, D., GUERRE, J.P., LEBLANC, P. and HICKMAN, C. (1998). "Radionuclide and radiation protection data handbook," Radiat. Prot. Dosim. **76**(1–2), 1–126.

DEL REGATO, J.A. (1985). *Radiological Physicists* (American Institute of Physics, New York).

DEL REGATO, J.A. (1996a). "The unfolding of American radiotherapy," Int. J. Radiat. Oncol. Biol. Phys. **35**(1), 5–14.

DEL REGATO, J.A. (1996b). "The international club of radiotherapists," Int. J. Radiat. Oncol. Biol. Phys. **35**(1), 21–26.

DEMPSEY, J.F., WILLIAMS, J.A., STUBBS, J.B., PATRICK, T.J. and WILLIAMSON, J.F. (1998). "Dosimetric properties of a novel brachytherapy balloon applicator for the treatment of malignant brain-tumor resection-cavity margins," Int. J. Radiat. Oncol. Biol. Phys. **42**(2), 421–429.

DOT (2006). U.S. Department of Transportation. *Transportation*. 49 CFR Parts 100–185 (revised and issued May 15) (U.S. Government Printing Office, Washington).

EDMONDS, C.J. and SMITH, T. (1986). "The long-term hazards of the treatment of thyroid cancer with radioiodine," Br. J. Radiol. **59**(697), 45–51.

EZZELL, G.A. (1995). "Commissioning of single stepping-source remote applicators," pages 557 to 576 in *Brachytherapy Physics*, Williamson, J.F., Thomadsen, B.R. and Nath, R., Eds. (Medical Physics Publishing Company, Madison, Wisconsin).

FAIRCHILD, R.G., BRILL, A.B. and ETTINGER, K.V. (1982). "Radiation enhancement with iodinated deoxyuridine," Invest. Radiol. **17**(4), 407–416.

FAIRCHILD, R.G., KALEF-ERZA, J., PACKER, S., WIELOPSKI, L., LASTER B.H., ROBERTSON, J.S., MAUSNER, L. and KANELLITSAS, C. (1987). "Samarium-145: A new brachytherapy source," Phys. Med. Biol. **32**(7), 847–858.

FISCHELL, T.A., KHARMA, B.K., FISCHELL, D.R., LOGES, P.G., COFFEY, C.W., II, DUGGAN, D.M. and NAFTILAN, A.J. (1994). "Low-dose beta-particle emission from stent wire results in complete, localized inhibition of smooth muscle cell proliferation," Circulation 90(6), 2956–2963.

FOLKERTS, K.H., FRANZ, A., KIEFER, A. and HENNERSDORF, G. (2002). "Radiation exposure of health personnel and patients in the heart catheterization laboratory during vascular brachytherapy," Z. Kardiol. 91(6), 493–502.

FREEMAN, L.M. and BLAUFOX, M.D., Eds. (1989). "Monoclonal antibodies I and II," Sem. Nucl. Med. 19(3), 157–246 and Nucl. Med. 19(4), 251–339.

FREEMAN, L.M. and BLAUFOX, M.D., Eds. (1992). "Radionuclide therapy of intractable bone pain," Sem. Nucl. Med. 22(1), 1–58.

GATES, V.L., CAREY, J.E., SIEGEL, J.A., KAMINSKI, M.S. and WAHL, R.L. (1998). "Nonmyeloablative ^{131}I anti-B1 radioimmunotherapy as outpatient therapy," J. Nucl. Med. 39(7), 1230–1236.

GEORGOPOULOS, M., ZEHETMAYER, M., RUHSWURM, I., TOMA-BSTAENDIG, S., SEGUR-ELTZ, N., SACU, S. and MENAPACE, R. (2003). "Tumor regression of uveal melanoma after ^{106}Ru brachytherapy of stereotactic radiotherapy with gamma knife or linear accelerator," Ophthalmologica 217(5), 315–319.

GLASGOW, G.P. (1995a). "Principles of remote afterloading devices," pages 485 to 502 in Brachytherapy Physics, Williamson J.F., Thomadsen B.T. and Nath R., Eds. (Medical Physics Publishing Company, Madison, Wisconsin).

GLASGOW, G.P. and CORRIGAN, K.W. (1995b). "Radiation design and control features of a hospital room for a low-dose-rate remote afterloading unit," Health Phys. 69(3), 415–419.

GLASGOW, G.P., BOURLAND, J.D., GRIGSBY, P.W., MELI, J.A. and WEAVER, K.A. (1993). Remote Afterloading Technology (American Institute of Physics, New York).

GLASSER, O., QUIMBY, E., TAYLOR, L.S., WEATHERWAX, J. and MORGAN, R. (1961). Physical Foundations of Radiology, 3rd ed. (Harper and Row, New York).

GOTTHARDT, M., BOERMANN, O.C., BEHR, T.M., BEHE, M.P. and OYEN, W.J.G. (2004). "Development and clinical application of peptide-based radiopharmaceuticals," Curr. Phar. Des. 10(24), 2951–2963.

GRANERO, D., PEREZ-CALATAYUD, J., BALLESTER, F., BOS, A.J.J. and VENSELAAR, J. (2006). "Broad-beam transmission data for new brachytherapy sources, ^{170}Tm and ^{169}Yb," Radiat. Prot. Dosim. 118(1), 11–15.

GRIGSBY, P.W., WILLIAMSON, J.F. and PEREZ, C.A. (1992). "Source configuration and dose rates for the selectron afterloading equipment for gynecologic applicators," Int. J. Radiat. Oncol. Biol. Phys. 24(2), 321–327.

GRIGSBY, P.W., SIEGEL, B.A., BAKER, S. and EICHLING, J.O. (2000). "Radiation exposure from outpatient radioactive iodine (^{131}I) therapy for thyroid carcinoma," JAMA **283**(17), 2272–2274.

GUNASEKERA, R., THOMSON, W. and HARDING, L. (1996). "Use of public transport by ^{131}I patients," (abstract) Nucl. Med. Commun. **17**, 275.

HALL, E.T. (1966). *The Hidden Dimension* (Doubleday Company, New York).

HANDELSMAN, D.J. and TURTLE, J.R. (1983). "Testicular damage after radioactive iodine (^{131}I) therapy for thyroid cancer," Clin. Endocrinol. **18**(5), 465–472.

HANSON, W.F. (1995). "Brachytherapy source strength: Quantities, units, and standards," pages 71 to 89 in *Brachytherapy Physics (1994 Summer School)*, Williamson J.F., Thomadsen B.R. and Nath, R., Eds. (Medical Physics Publishing, Madison, Wisconsin).

HARBERT, J.C. (1987). *Nuclear Medicine Therapy* (Thieme Medical Publishers, New York).

HARBERT, J.C. and WELLS, N. (1974). "Radiation exposure of the family of radioactive patients," J. Nucl. Med. **15**(10), 887–888.

HENSCHKE, U.K., HILARIS, B.S. and MAHAN, G.D. (1963). "Afterloading in interstitial and intracavitary radiation therapy," Am. J. Roentgenol. Radium Ther. Nucl. Med. **90**, 386–395.

HERBA, M.J., ILLESCAS, F.F., THIRLWELL, M.P., BOOS, G.J., ROSENTHALL, L., ATRI, M. and BRET, P.M. (1988). "Hepatic malignancies: Improved treatment with intraarterial ^{90}Y," Radiology **169**(2), 311–314.

HILARIS, B.S., HOLT, G.J. and ST. GERMAIN, J. (1975). *The Use of ^{125}I for Interstitial Implants*, DHEW/FDA 76-8022 (U.S. Food and Drug Administration, Rockville, Maryland).

HODT, H.J., SINCLAIR, W.K. and SMITHERES, D.W. (1952). "A gun for interstitial implantation of radioactive gold grains," Brit. J. Radiol. **25**(296), 419–421.

HOLM, H.H., JUUL, N., PEDERSON, J.F., HANSEN, H. and STROYER, I. (1983). "Transperineal ^{125}I seed implantation in prostatic cancer guided by transrectal ultrasonography," J. Urol. **130**, 283–286.

HOSAIN, F. and HOSAIN, P. (1978). "Selection of radionuclides for therapy," pages 33 to 43 in *Therapy in Nuclear Medicine*, Spencer, R.P., Ed. (Grune and Stratton, New York).

HSIAO, E., HUYNH, T., MANSBERG, R., BAUTOVICH, G. and ROACH, P. (2004). "Diagnostic ^{123}I scintigraphy to assess potential breast uptake of ^{131}I before radioiodine therapy in a postpartum woman with thyroid cancer," Clin. Nucl. Med. **29**(8), 498–501.

HUNDAHL, S.A., FLEMING, I.D., FREMGEN, A.M. and MENCK, H.R. (1998). "A national cancer data base report on 53,856 cases of thyroid carcinoma treated in the U.S., 1985-1995," Cancer **83**(12), 2638–2648.

HUSTINX, R., YEUNG, H., PAULUS, P., MACAPINLAC, H., RIGO, P. and LARSON, S.(1996). "Clinical PET in oncology," Eur. J. Nucl. Med. **23**(12), 1641–1974

HYER, S., VINI, L., O'CONNELL, M., PRATT, B. and HARMER, C. (2002). "Testicular dose and fertility in men following ^{131}I therapy for thyroid cancer," Clin. Endocrinol. **56**(6), 755–758.

ICRP (1983). International Commission on Radiological Protection. *Cost-Benefit Analysis in the Optimization of Radiation Safety*, ICRP Publication 37, Ann. ICRP **10**(2/3) (Elsevier Science, New York).

ICRP (1989). International Commission on Radiological Protection. *Optimization and Decision-Making in Radiological Protection*, ICRP Publication 55, Ann. ICRP **20**(1) (Elsevier Science, New York).

ICRP (1991). International Commission on Radiological Protection. *1990 Recommendations of the International Commission on Radiological Protection—Users' Edition*, ICRP Publication 60 Ann. ICRP **21**(1-3) (Elsevier Science, New York).

ICRP (1993). International Commission on Radiological Protection. *Summary of the Current ICRP Principles for Protection of the Patient in Nuclear Medicine*, # (Elsevier Science, New York).

ICRU (1985). International Commission on Radiation Units and Measurements. *Dose and Volume Specification for Reporting Intracavitary Therapy in Gynecology*, ICRU Report 38 (Oxford University Press, Cary, North Carolina).

ICRU (1989). International Commission on Radiation Units and Measurements. *Tissue Substitutes in Radiation Dosimetry and Measurement*, ICRU Report 44 (Oxford University Press, Cary, North Carolina).

ICRU (1993). International Commission on Radiation Units and Measurements. *Quantities and Units in Radiation Protection Dosimetry*, ICRU Report 51 (Oxford University Press, Cary, North Carolina).

ICRU (1997). International Commission on Radiation Units and Measurements. *Dose and Volume Specification for Reporting Interstitial Therapy*, ICRU Report 58 (Oxford University Press, Cary, North Carolina).

ICRU (1998a). International Commission on Radiation Units and Measurements. *Fundamental Quantities and Units for Ionizing Radiation*, ICRU Report 60 (Oxford University Press, Cary, North Carolina).

ICRU (1998b). International Commission on Radiation Units and Measurements. *Conversion Coefficients for Use in Radiological Protection Against External Radiation*, ICRU Report 57 (Oxford University Press, Cary, North Carolina).

ICRU (2004). International Commission on Radiation Units and Measurements. *Dosimetry of Beta Rays and Low-Energy Photons for Brachytherapy with Sealed Sources*, ICRU Report 72 (Oxford University Press, Cary, North Carolina).

JACOBSON, A.P., PLATO, P.A. and TOEROEK, D. (1978). "Contamination of the home environment by patients treated with [131]I: Initial results," Am. J. Public Health **68**(3), 228–230.

JHANWAR, Y. and DIVGI, C. R. (2005). "Current status of therapy of solid tumors," J. Nucl. Med **46** (Suppl. 1), S141–S150.

JOLIOT, F. and CURIE, I. (1934). "Artificial production of a new kind of radio-element," Nature **133**, 201.

KAPLAN, W.D., ZIMMERMAN, R.E., BLOOMER, W.D., KNAPP, R.C. and ADELSTEIN, S.J. (1981). "Therapeutic intraperitoneal ^{32}P: A clinical assessment of the dynamics of distribution," Radiology **138**, 683–688.

KRAMER, K. and CHEUNG, N.K. (2001). "Antibody-based diagnostic and therapeutic innovations for human cancer," Compr. Ther. **27**(3), 183–194.

KUBO, H.D., GLASGOW, G.P., PETHEL, T.D., THOMADSEN, B.R. and WILLIAMSON, J.F. (1998). "High dose-rate brachytherapy treatment delivery: Report of the AAPM Radiation Therapy Committee Task Group No. 59," Med. Phys. **25**(4), 375–403.

KUTCHER, G.J., COICA, L., GILLIN, M., HANSON, W.F., LEIBEL, S., MORTON, R.J., PALTA, J.R., PURDY, J.A., REINSTEIN, L.E., SVENSSON, G.K., WELLER, M. and WINGFIELD, L. (1994). "Comprehensive QA for radiation oncology: Report of the AAPM Radiation Therapy Committee Task Group 40," Med. Phys. **21**(4), 581–618.

LASHFORD, L.Z., DAVIES, A.G., RICHARDSON, R.B., BOURNE, S.P., BULLIMORE, J.A., ECKERT, H., KEMSHEAD, J.T. and COAKHAM, H.B. (1988). "A pilot study of ^{131}I monoclonal antibodies in the therapy of leptomeningeal tumors," Cancer **61**, 857–868.

LAUGHLIN, J.S., VACIRCA, S.J. and DUPLISSEY, J.R. (1968). "Exposure of embalmers and physicians by radioactive cadavers," Health Phys. **15**(5), 451–455.

LAWRENCE, E.O. and COOKSEY, D. (1936). "On the apparatus for the multiple acceleration of light ions to high speeds," Phys. Rev. **50**(12), 1131–1140.

LAWRENCE, E.O. and LIVINGSTON, M.S. (1934). "The multiple acceleration of ions to very high speeds," Phys. Rev. **45**(9), 608–612.

LIM, L., GIBBS, P., YIP, D., SHAPIRO, J.D., DOWLING, R., SMITH, D., LITTLE, A., BAILEY, W. and LICHTENSTEIN, M. (2005). "Prospective study of treatment with selective internal radiation therapy spheres in patients with unresectable primary or secondary hepatic malignancies," Intern. Med. J. **35**(4), 222–227.

LING, C.C. (1992). "Permanent implants using ^{198}Au, ^{103}Pd, and ^{125}I: Radiobiological considerations based on the linear quadratic model," Int. J. Radiat. Oncol. Biol. Phys. **23**(1), 81–87.

LIVINGOOD, J.J. and SEABORG, G.T. (1938). "Radioactive iodine isotopes," Phys. Rev. **53**(2), 1015.

LOEVINGER, R. and FEITELBERG, S. (1955). "Using bremsstrahlung detection by a scintillator for simplified beta counting," Nucleonics **13**(4), 42–45.

LYMPEROPOULOU, G., PAPAGIANNIS, P., SAKELLIOU, L., GEORGIOU, E., HOURDAKIS, C.J. and BALTAS, D. (2006). "Comparison of radiation shielding requirements for HDR brachytherapy using ^{169}Yb and ^{192}Ir sources," Med. Phys **33**(7), 2541–2547.

MACEY, D.J., WILLIAMS, L.E., BREITZ, H.B., LIU, A., JOHNSON, T.K. and ZANZONICO, P.B. (2001). "A primer for radioimmunotherapy and radionuclide therapy," Report No. 71 (American Association of Physicists in Medicine, College Park, Maryland).

MANHATTAN (1946). Manhattan Project. "Availability of radioactive isotopes: Announcement from headquarters, Manhattan Project, Washington, D.C.," Science, **103**(2685), 697–716.

MARUYAMA, Y., WIERZBICKI, J.G., TYURIN, B.M. and KANETA, K. (1997). "Californium-252 neutron brachytherapy," pages 649 to 687 in *Principles and Practice of Brachytherapy*, Nag, S. and James, A.G., Eds. (Futura Publishing Company, Inc., Armonk, New York).

MASON, D.L., BATTISTA, J.J., BARNETT, R.B. and PORTER, A.T. (1992). "Ytterbium-169: Calculated physical properties of a new radiation source for brachytherapy," Med. Phys. **19**(3), 695–703.

MASSULLO, V.M., TIERSTEIN, P.S., JANI, S.K., RUSSO, R.J., GUARNERI, E.M., JIN, H., SCHATZ, R.A., MORRIS, N.B., STEUTERMAN, S., POPMA, J.J., MINTZ, G.S., LEON, M.B. and TRIPURANENI, P. (1996). "Endovascular brachytherapy to inhibit coronary artery restenosis: An introduction to the SCRIPPS coronary radiation to inhibit proliferation post stenting trial," Int. J. Radiat. Oncol. Biol. Phys. **36**(4) 973–975.

MATHIEU, I., CAUSSIN, J., SMEESTERS, P., WAMBERSIE, A. and BECKERS, C. (1997). "Doses in family members after ^{131}I treatment," Lancet **350**(9084), 1074–1075.

MATHIEU, I., CAUSSIN, J., SMEESTERS. P., WAMBERSIE, A. and BECKERS, C. (1999). "Recommended restrictions after ^{131}I therapy: Measured doses in family members," Health Phys. **76**(2), 129–136.

MCDEVITT, M.R., SGOUROS, G., FINN, R.D., HUMM, J.J., JURCIC, J.G., LARSON, S.M. and SCHEINBERG, D.A. (1998). "Radioimmunotherapy with alpha-emitting nuclides," Eur. J. Nucl. Med. **25**(9), 1341–1351.

MCDEVITT, M.R., FINN, R.D., SGOUROS, G., MA, D. and SCHEINBERG, D.A. (1999). "An [225]Ac/[213]Bi generator system for therapeutic clinical applications: Construction and operation," Appl. Radiat. Isot. **50**(5), 895–904.

MELIA, B.M., ABRAMSON, D.H., ALBERT, D. M., BOLDT, H.C., EARLE, J.D., HANSON, W.F., MONTAGUE, P., MOY, C.S., SCHACHAT, A.P., SIMPSON, E.R., STRAATSMA, B.R., VINE, A.K. and WEINGEIST, T.A. (2001). "Collaborative ocular melanoma study (COMS) randomized trial of [25]I brachytherapy for medium choroidal melanoma: I. Visual acuity after 3 years, COMS Report No. 16," Ophthalmol. **108**(2), 348–366.

MEREDITH, R.F. and KNOX, S.J. (2006). "Clinical development of radioimmunotherapy for B-cell non-Hodgkin's lymphoma," Int. J. Radiat. Oncol. Biol. Phys. **66** (Suppl. 2), S15–S22.

MERRICK, G.S., BUTLER, W.M., DORSEY, A.T, LIEF, J.H. and BENSON, M.L. (2000). "Seed fixity in the prostate/periprostatic region following brachytherapy," Int. J. Radiat. Oncol. Biol. Phys. **46**(1), 215–220.

MILLER, K.M. (1992). "External radiation doses in a household from a patient receiving a therapeutic amount of ^{131}I," pages 1 to 25 in *Report of the Environmental Measurement Laboratory*, EML-547 (U.S. Department of Energy, New York).

MURTHY, R., NUNEZ, R., SZKLARUK, J., ERWIN, W., MADOFF, D.C., GUPTA, S., AHRAR, K., WALLACE, M.J., COHEN, A., COLDWELL, D.M., KENNEDY, A.S. and HICKS, M.E. (2005a). "Yttrium-90 microsphere therapy for hepatic malignancy: Devices, indications, technical considerations, and potential complications," Radiographics **25** (Suppl. 1) S41–S55

MURTHY, R., HANAVAZ, S.G., NAIK, M., GOPI, S. and REDDY, V.A. (2005b). "Ruthenium-106 plaque brachytherapy for the treatment of diffuse choroidal haemangioma in Sturge-Weber syndrome," Indian J. Ophthalmol. **53**(4), 274–275.

MYERS, W.G. (1948). "Applications of artificially radioactive isotopes in therapy," Am. J. Roentgenol. Rad. Ther. **60**(6), 816–823.

MYERS, C.A. and ABRAMSON, D.H. (1988). "Radiation protection: Choroidal mclanoma and ^{125} iodine plaques," J. Opthalmic Nurs. Technol. **7**(3), 103–107.

NAG, S., VIVEKANANDAM, S. and MARTINEZ-MONGE, R. (1997). "Pulmonary embolization of permanently implanted radioactive ^{103}Pd seeds for carcinoma of the prostate," Int. J. Radiat. Oncol. Biol. Phys. **39**(3) 667–670.

NAS/NRC (1990). National Academy of Sciences/National Research Council. *Health Effects of Exposure to Low Levels of Ionizing Radiation*, Report of the Committee on the Biological Effects of Ionizing Radiation (BEIR V) (National Academy Press, Washington).

NAS/NRC (2006). National Academy of Sciences/National Research Council. *Health Risks from Exposure to Low Levels of Ionizing Radiation: BEIR VII Phase 2*, Report of the Committee to Assess Health Risks from Exposure to Low Levels of Ionizing Radiation (BEIR VII) (National Academy Press, Washington).

NATH, R. and ROBERTS, K.B. (1996). "Vascular irradiation for the prevention of restenosis after angioplasty: A new application for radiotherapy," Int. J. Radiat. Oncol. Biol. Phys. **36**(4), 977–979.

NATH, R., PESCHEL, R.E., PARK, C.H. and FISCHER J.J. (1988). "Development of an ^{241}Am applicator for intracavitary irradiation of gynecologic cancers," Int. J. Radiat. Oncol. Biol. Phys. **14**(5), 969–978.

NATH, R., ANDERSON, L.L., LUXTON, G., WEAVER, K.A., WILLIAMSON, J.F. and MEIGOONI, A.S. (1995). "Dosimetry of interstitial brachytherapy sources: Recommendations of the AAPM Radiation Therapy Committee Task Group No. 43," Med. Phys. **22**(2), 209–234.

NATH, R., ANDERSON, L.L., MELI, J.A., OLCH, A.J., STITT, J.A. and WILLIAMSON, J.F. (1997). "Code of practice for brachytherapy physics: Report of the AAPM Radiation Therapy Committee Task Group No. 56," Med. Phys. **24**(10), 1557–1648.

NCRP (1970). National Council on Radiation Protection and Measurements. *Precautions in the Management of Patients Who Have Received Therapeutic Amounts of Radionuclides*, NCRP Report No. 37 (National

Council on Radiation Protection and Measurements, Bethesda, Maryland).

NCRP (1976). National Council on Radiation Protection and Measurements. *Structural Shielding Design and Evaluation for Medical Use of X Rays and Gamma Rays of Energies Up to 10 MeV*, NCRP Report No. 49 (National Council on Radiation Protection and Measurements, Bethesda, Maryland).

NCRP (1983). National Council on Radiation Protection and Measurements. *Operational Radiation Safety – Training*, NCRP Report No. 71 (National Council on Radiation Protection and Measurements, Bethesda, Maryland).

NCRP (1987). National Council on Radiation Protection and Measurements. *Recommendations on Limits for Exposure to Ionizing Radiation*, NCRP Report No. 91 (National Council on Radiation Protection and Measurements, Bethesda, Maryland).

NCRP (1989). National Council on Radiation Protection and Measurements. *Radiation Protection for Medical and Allied Health Personnel*, NCRP Report No. 105 (National Council on Radiation Protection and Measurements, Bethesda, Maryland).

NCRP (1990). National Council on Radiation Protection and Measurements. *Implementation of the Principle of As Low As Reasonably Achievable (ALARA) for Medical and Dental Personnel*, NCRP Report No. 107 (National Council on Radiation Protection and Measurements, Bethesda, Maryland).

NCRP (1992a). National Council on Radiation Protection and Measurements. *Calibration of Survey Instruments Used in Radiation Protection for the Assessment of Ionizing Radiation Fields and Radioactive Surface Contamination*, NCRP Report No. 112 (National Council on Radiation Protection and Measurements, Bethesda, Maryland).

NCRP (1992b). National Council on Radiation Protection and Measurements. *Maintaining Radiation Protection Records*, NCRP Report No. 114 (National Council on Radiation Protection and Measurements, Bethesda, Maryland).

NCRP (1993a). National Council on Radiation Protection and Measurements. *Risk Estimates for Radiation Protection*, NCRP Report No. 115 (National Council on Radiation Protection and Measurements, Bethesda, Maryland).

NCRP (1993b). National Council on Radiation Protection and Measurements. *Limitation of Exposure to Ionizing Radiation*, NCRP Report No. 116 (National Council on Radiation Protection and Measurements, Bethesda, Maryland).

NCRP (1994). National Council on Radiation Protection and Measurements. *Considerations Regarding the Unintended Radiation Exposure of the Embryo, Fetus or Nursing Child*, NCRP Commentary No. 9 (National Council on Radiation Protection and Measurements, Bethesda, Maryland).

NCRP (1995a). National Council on Radiation Protection and Measurements. *Dose Limits for Individuals Who Receive Exposure from*

Radionuclide Therapy Patients, NCRP Commentary No. 11 (National Council on Radiation Protection and Measurements, Bethesda, Maryland).

NCRP (1995b). National Council on Radiation Protection and Measurements. *Use of Personal Monitors to Estimate Effective Dose Equivalent and Effective Dose to Workers for External Exposure to Low-LET Radiation*, NCRP Report No. 122 (National Council on Radiation Protection and Measurements, Bethesda, Maryland).

NCRP (1996). National Council on Radiation Protection and Measurements. *Sources and Magnitude of Occupational and Public Exposures from Nuclear Medicine Procedures*, NCRP Report No. 124 (National Council on Radiation Protection and Measurements, Bethesda, Maryland).

NCRP (1998). National Council on Radiation Protection and Measurements. *Operational Radiation Safety Program*, NCRP Report No. 127 (National Council on Radiation Protection and Measurements, Bethesda, Maryland).

NCRP (1999a). National Council on Radiation Protection and Measurements. *The Effects of Pre- and Postconception Exposure to Radiation*, NCRP Annual Meeting Proceedings No. 19 (National Council on Radiation Protection and Measurements, Bethesda, Maryland).

NCRP (1999b). National Council on Radiation Protection and Measurements. *Radiation Protection in Medicine: Contemporary Issues*, NCRP Annual Meeting Proceedings No. 21 (National Council on Radiation Protection and Measurements, Bethesda, Maryland).

NCRP (2000). National Council on Radiation Protection and Measurements. *Operational Radiation Safety Training*, NCRP Report No. 134 (National Council on Radiation Protection and Measurements, Bethesda, Maryland).

NCRP (2003). National Council on Radiation Protection and Measurements. *Management Techniques for Laboratories and Other Small Institutional Generators to Minimize Off-Site Disposal of Low-Level Radioactive Waste*, NCRP Report No. 143 (National Council on Radiation Protection and Measurements, Bethesda, Maryland).

NCRP (2004a). National Council on Radiation Protection and Measurements. *Recent Applications of the NCRP Public Dose Limit Recommendation for Ionizing Radiation*, NCRP Statement No. 10 (National Council on Radiation Protection and Measurements, Bethesda, Maryland).

NCRP (2004b). National Council on Radiation Protection and Measurements. *Structural Shielding Design for Medical X-Ray Imaging Facilities*, NCRP Report No. 147 (National Council on Radiation Protection and Measurements, Bethesda, Maryland).

NCRP (2005). National Council on Radiation Protection and Measurements. *Structural Shielding Design and Evaluation for Megavoltage X- and Gamma-Ray Radiotherapy Facilities*, NCRP Report No. 151 (National Council on Radiation Protection and Measurements, Bethesda, Maryland).

NEBLETT, D.L. and WESICK, J.S. (1995). "Quality assurance of computer-assisted treatment planning," pages 253 to 264 in *Brachytherapy Physics*, Williamson, J.F., Thomadsen, B.R. and Nath, R., Eds. (Medical Physics Publishing Company, Madison, Wisconsin).

NIST (2001). National Institute of Standards and Technology. *Calibration of X-Ray and Gamma-Ray Measuring Instruments*, SP 250-58 (National Technical Information Service, Springfield, Virginia).

NRC (1987). U.S. Nuclear Regulatory Commission. *Medical Use of By-Product Material*, 35 CFR 10(1) (U.S. Government Printing Office, Washington).

NRC (1988). U.S. Nuclear Regulatory Commission. *Standards for Protection Against Radiation*, 20 CFR 10(1) (U.S. Government Printing Office, Washington).

NRC (1991). U.S. Nuclear Regulatory Commission. *Quality Management Program and Misadministrations*, 56 FR 34104 (U.S. Government Printing Office, Washington).

NRC (1993a). U.S. Nuclear Regulatory Commission. *Release of Patients after Brachytherapy Treatment with Remote Afterloading Devices*, NRC Bulletin 93-01 (U.S. Government Printing Office, Washington).

NRC (1993b). U.S. Nuclear Regulatory Commission. *Loss of an Iridium-192 Source and Therapy Misadministration at Indiana Regional Cancer Center, Indiana, Pennsylvania on November 16, 1992*, NUREG-1480 (U.S. Government Printing Office, Washington).

NRC (1997a). U.S. Nuclear Regulatory Commission. *Regulatory Analysis on Criteria for the Release of Patients Administered Radioactive Material*, NUREG-1492 (U.S. Government Printing Office, Washington).

NRC (1997b). U.S. Nuclear Regulatory Commission. *Release of Patients Administered Radioactive Materials*, Regulatory Guide 8.39 (U.S. Government Printing Office, Washington).

NRC (2002). U.S. Nuclear Regulatory Commission. *Program Specific Guidance About Medical Use Licenses – Final Report*, NUREG-1556, Vol. 9 (U.S. Government Printing Office, Washington).

NRC (2004). U.S. Nuclear Regulatory Commission. *Report to Congress on Abnormal Occurrences Fiscal Year 2003: Dissemination of Information*, 69 FR 24688 (U.S. Government Printing Office, Washington).

NRC (2005). U.S. Nuclear Regulatory Commission. *Consolidated Guidance About Materials Licenses: Program-Specific Guidance About Medical Use Licenses - Final Report*, NUREG-1556, Vol. 9 (U.S. Government Printing Office, Washington).

PACINI, F., GASPERI, M., FUGAZZOLA, L., CECCARELLI, C., LIPPI, F., CENTONI, R., MARTINO, E. and PINCHERA, A. (1994). "Testicular function in patients with differentiated thyroid carcinoma treated with radioiodine," J. Nucl. Med. **35**(9), 1418–1422.

PANDIT-TASKAR, N., HAMLIN P.A., REYES S., LARSON, S.M. and DIVGI C.R. (2003). "New strategies in radioimmunotherapy for lymphoma," Curr. Oncol. Rep. **5**(5), 354–371.

PANDIT-TASKAR, N., BATRAKI, M. and DIVGI, C.R. (2004). "Radiopharmaceutical therapy for palliation of bone pain from osseous metastases," J. Nucl. Med. 45(8), 1358–1365.

PARYANI, S.B., SCOTT, W.P. and WELLS, J.W., JR. (1994). "Management of pterygium with surgery and radiation therapy. The North Florida pterygium study group," Int. J. Radiat. Oncol. Biol. Phys. 28(1), 101–103.

PATERSON, R. (1934). "A dosage system for gamma ray therapy," Brit. J. Radiol. 7, 592.

PATERSON, R., PARKER, H.M. and SPIERS, F.W. (1936). "A system of dosage for cylindrical distributions of radium," Brit. J. Radiol. 9, 487.

PENTLOW, K.S., GRAHAM, M.C., LAMBRECHT, R.M., CHEUNG, N.K. and LARSON, S.M. (1991). "Quantitative imaging of [124]I using positron emission tomography with applications to radioimmunodiagnosis and radioimmunotherapy," Med. Phys. 18(3), 357–366.

PENTLOW, K.S., GRAHAM, M.C., LAMBRECHT, R.M., DAGHIGHIAN, F., BACHARACH, S.L., BENDRIEM, B., FINN, R.D., JORDAN, K., KALAIGIAN, H., KARP, J.S., ROBESON, W.R. and LARSON, S.M. (1996). "Quantitative imaging of [124]I with PET," J. Nucl. Med. 37(9), 1557–1562.

PERERA, H., WILLIAMSON, J.F., LI, Z., MISHRA, V. and MEIGOONI, A.S. (1994). "Dosimetric characteristics, air-kerma strength calibration and verification of Monte Carlo simulation for a new [169]Yb brachytherapy source," Int. J. Radiat. Oncol. Biol. Phys. 28(4), 953–971.

PIERMATTEI, A., ARCOVITO, G., AZARIO, L., ROSSI, G., SORIANI, A. and MONTEMAGGI, P. (1992). "Experimental dosimetry of [169]Yb seeds prototype 6 for brachytherapy treatment," Physica Medica 8, 163–169.

PIERMATTEI, A., AZARIO, L. and MONTEMAGGI, A. (1995). "Implantation guidelines for [169]Yb seed interstitial treatments," Phys. Med. Biol. 40(8), 1331–1338.

PIERQUIN, B., WILSON, J.F. and CHASSAGNE, D., Eds. (1987). Modern Brachytherapy (Year Book Medical Publishers, New York).

POCHIN, E.E. and KERMODE, J.C. (1975). "Protection problems in radionuclide therapy: The patient as a gamma-radiation source," Br. J. Radiol. 48(568), 299–305.

PORTER, A.T., SCRIMGER, J.W. and POCHA, J.S. (1988). "Remote interstitial afterloading in cancer of the prostate: Preliminary experience with the MicroSelectron," Int. J. Radiat. Oncol. Biol. Phys. 14(3), 571–575.

QUE, W. (2001). "Radiation safety issues regarding the cremation of the body of an ^{125}I prostate implant patient," J. Appl. Clin. Med. Phys. 2(3), 174–177.

QUIMBY, E.H. (1931). "Comparison of various sources of interstitial irradiation," Am J. Roentgenol. Radium Ther. 17, 449–470.

QUIMBY, E. (1935). "Physical factors in interstitial radium therapy," Am. J. Roentgenol. & Radium Ther. 33(3), 306–316.

QUIMBY, E.H. (1948). "Fifty years of radium," Am. J. Roentgenol. **60**, 723–727.

QUIMBY, E. and MACOMB, W.S. (1937). "Further studies on the rate of recovery of the human skin from the effects of roentgen or gamma ray irradiation," Radiology **29**, 305–312.

QUIMBY, E.H., FEITELBERG, S. and GROSS, W. (1970). *Radioactive Nuclides in Medicine and Biology* (Lea and Febiger, Philadelphia).

RUSSELL, W.L. (1977). "Mutation frequencies in female mice and the estimation of genetic hazards of radiation in women," Proc. Natl. Acad. Sci. **74**(8), 3523–3527.

RUSSELL, W.L. and KELLY, E.M. (1982). "Mutation frequencies in male mice and the estimation of genetic hazards of radiation in men," Proc. Natl. Acad. Sci. **79**(2), 542–544.

RUTAR, F.J., AUGUSTINE, S.C., COLCHER, D., SIEGEL, J.A., JACOBSON, D.A., TEMPERO, M.A., DUKAT, V.J., HOHENSTEIN, M.A., GOBAR, L.S. and VOSE, J.M. (2001a). "Outpatient treatment with ^{131}I anti-B1 antibody: Radiation exposure to family members," J. Nucl. Med. **42**(6), 907–915.

RUTAR, F.J., AUGUSTINE, S.C., KAMINSKI, M.S., WAHL, R.L., SIEGEL, J.A. and COLCHER, D. (2001b). "Feasibility and safety of outpatient Bexxar therapy (Tositumomab and [131]I Tositumomab) for non-Hodgkin's lymphoma based on radiation doses to family members," Clin. Lymphoma **2**(3), 164–172.

RYAN, M.T., SPICER, K.M., FREI-LAHR, D., SAMEI, E., FREY, G.D., HARGROVE, H. and BLOODWORTH, G. (2000). "Health physics consequences of out-patient treatment of non-Hodgkin's lymphoma with ^{131}I-radiolabeled anti-B1 antibody," Oper. Radiat. Safety **79**(5), S52–S55.

SALEM, R. and THURSTON, K.G. (2006). "'Radioembolization' with ^{90}Y microspheres: A state-of-the-art brachytherapy treatment for primary and secondary liver malignancies: Part 1: Technical and methodologic considerations," J. Vasc. Interv. Radiol. **17**, 1251–1278.

SAMUELS, M., PESCHEL, R.E., PAPADOPOULOS, D., DOWLING, S., HAFFTY, B., NATH, R., CHAMBERS, J., CHAMBERS, S., KOHORN, E., SCHWARTZ, P.E. and FISCHER, J.J. (1991). "A feasibility study of intracavitary [241]Am for recurrent pelvic malignancies," Endocurie Hypertherm. Oncol. **7**, 131–137.

SARKAR, S.D., BEIERWALTES, W.H., GILL, S.P. and COWLEY, B.J. (1976). "Subsequent fertility and birth histories of children and adolescents treated with ^{131}I for thyroid cancer," J. Nucl. Med. **17**(6), 460–464.

SCHLUMBERGER, M., DEVATHAIRE, F., CECCARELLI, C., DELISLE, M.J., FRANCESE, C., COUETTE, J.E., PINCHERA, A. and PARMENTIER, C. (1996). "Exposure to radioactive ^{131}I for scintigraphy or therapy does not preclude pregnancy in thyroid cancer patients," J. Nucl. Med. **37**(4), 606–612.

SCHODER, H., ERDI, Y.E., LARSON, S.M. and YEUNG, H.W. (2003). "PET/CT: A new imaging technology in nuclear medicine," Eur. J. Nucl. Med. Mol. Imaging 30(10), 1419–1437.

SCHOPOHL, B., LIERMANN, D., POHLIT, L.J., HEYD, R., STRASSMANN, G., BAUERSACHS, R., SCHULTE-HUERMANN, D., RAHL, C.G., MANEGOLD, K.II., KOLLATH, J. and BOTTCHER, H.D. (1996). "Iridium-192 endovascular brachytherapy for avoidance of intimal hyperplasia after percutaneous transluminal angioplasty and stent implantation in peripheral vessels: 6 years of experience," Int. J. Radiat. Oncol. Biol. Phys. 36(4), 835–840.

SEPHTON, R., DAS, K.R., COLES, J., TOYE, W. and PINDER, P. (1999). "Local shielding of high dose rate brachytherapy in an operating theatre," Aust. Phys. Eng. Sci. Med. 22(3), 113–117.

SGOUROS, G. (2005). "Dosimetry of internal emitters," J. Nucl. Med. 46 (Suppl. 1), S18–S27.

SGOUROS, G., BALLANGRUD, A.M., JURCIC, J.G., MCDEVITT, M.R., HUMM, J.L., ERDI, Y.E., MEHTA, B.M., FINN, R.D., LARSON, S.M. and SCHEINBERG, D.A. (1999). "Pharmacokinetics and dosimetry of an alpha-particle emitter labeled antibody: ^{213}Bi-HuM195 (anti-CD33) in patients with leukemia," J. Nucl. Med. 40(11), 1935–1946.

SGOUROS, G., KOLBERT, K.S., SHEIKH, A., PENTLOW, K.S., MUN, E.F., BARTH, A., ROBBINS, R.J. and LARSON, S.M. (2004). "Patient-specific dosimetry for ^{131}I thyroid cancer therapy using ^{124}I PET and 3-dimensional dosimetry (3D-ID) software," J. Nucl. Med. 45(8), 1366–1372.

SIEGEL, J.A. (1998). "Revised Nuclear Regulatory Commission regulations for release of patients administered radioactive materials: Outpatient ^{131}I anti-B1 therapy," J. Nucl. Med. 39(8), S28–S33.

SIEGEL, J. (2004). Guide for Diagnostic Nuclear Medicine and Radiopharmaceutical Therapy (Society of Nuclear Medicine, Reston, Virginia).

SIEGEL, J.A. and RUTAR, F.J. (2002). "Possibility of internal contamination from radionuclide therapy patients released according to 10 CFR 35.75," Radiat. Prot. Manage. 19(1), 15–18.

SIEGEL, J.A., THOMAS, S.R., STUBBS, J.B., STAABIN, M.G., HAYS, M.T., KORAL, K.F., ROBERTSON, J.S., HOWELL, R.W., WESSELS, B.W., FISHER, D.R., WEBER, D.A. and BRILL, A.B. (1999). "MIRD Pamphlet 16: Techniques for quantitative radiopharmaceutical biodistribution data acquisition and analysis for use in human radiation dose estimates," J. Nucl. Med. 40(2) S37–S61.

SIEVERT, R.M. (1921). "Die intensitatsverteilung der primaren-strahlung in der Nahe medizinischer radiumpraparate," Acta Radiologica. 1, 89–128.

SINCLAIR, W.K. (1952). "Artificial sources for interstitial therapy," Br. J. Radiol. 25(296), 417–419.

SMATHERS, S., WALLNER, K., KORSSJOEN, T., BERGSAGEL, C., HUDSON, R.H., SUTLIEF, S. and BLASKO, J. (1999). "Radiation safety parameters following prostate brachytherapy," Int. J. Radiat. Oncol. Biol. Phys. **45**(2), 397–399.

SPARKS, R.B., SIEGEL, J.A. and WAHL, R.L. (1998). "The need for better methods to determine release criteria for patients administered radioactive material," Health Phys. **75**(4), 385–388.

SPENCER, R.P. (1978). "Nuclear medicine and therapy: A reorientation to specificity and beta-ray generators," pages 3 to 15 in *Therapy in Nuclear Medicine*, Spencer, R.P., Ed. (Grune and Stratton, New York).

SPITZWEG, C. and MORRIS, J.C. (2002). "The sodium iodide symporter: Its pathophysiological and therapeutic implications," Clin. Endocrinol. **57**(5), 559–574.

ST. GERMAIN, J. (1995). "Radiation monitoring with reference to the medical environment," Health Phys. **69**(5), 728–749.

STRZELCZYK, J. and SAFADI, R. (2004). "Radiation safety considerations in gliasite ^{125}I brain implant procedures," Health Phys. **86** (Suppl. 2), S120–S123.

STUBBS, R.S., CANNAN, R.J. and MITCHELL, A.W. (2001). "Selective internal radiation therapy with ^{90}Y microspheres for extensive colorectal liver metastases," J. Gastrointest. Surg. **5**(3), 294–302.

STUTZ, M., PETRIKAS, J., RASLOWSKY, M., LEE, P., GUREL, M. and MORAN, B. (2003). "Seed loss through the urinary tract after prostate brachytherapy: Examining the role of cystoscopy and urine straining post implant," Med. Phys. **30**(10), 2695–2698.

SUIT, H.D., MOORE, E.B., FLETCHER, G.H. and WORSNOP, R. (1963). "Modification of the Fletcher ovoid system for afterloading, using standard-sized radium tubes (milligram and microgram)," Radiology **81**, 126–131.

TEIRSTEIN, P.S., MASSULLO, V., JANI, S., POPMA, J.J., MINTZ, G.S., RUSSO, R.J., SCHATZ, R.A., GUARNERI, E.M., STEUTERMAM, S., MORRIS, N.B., LEON, M.B. and TRIPURANENI, P. (1997). "Catheter-based radiotherapy to inhibit restenosis after coronary stenting," N. Engl. J. Med. **336**(24), 1697–1703.

THOMADSEN, B.R. (1995). "Clinical implementation of remote-afterloading interstitial brachytherapy," pages 679 to 698 in *Brachytherapy Physics*, Williamson, J.F., Thomadsen, B.R. and Nath, R., Eds. (Medical Physics Publishing Company, Madison, Wisconsin).

THOMADSEN, B., LIN, S.W., LAEMMRICH, P., WALLER, T., CHENG, A., CALDWELL, B., RANKIN, R. and STITT, J. (2003), "Analysis of treatment delivery errors in brachytherapy using formal risk analysis techniques," Int. J. Radiat. Oncol. Biol. Phys. **57**, 1492–1508.

UNGER, L.M. and TRUBEY, D.K. (1982). *Specific Gamma-Ray Dose Constants for Nuclides Important to Dosimetry and Radiological Assessment*, ORNL/RSIC-45/R1 (Oak Ridge National Laboratory, Oak Ridge, Tennessee).

UNSCEAR (1977). United National Scientific Committee on the Effects of Atomic Radiation. *Sources and Effects of Ionizing Radiation, UNSCEAR 1977 Report to the General Assembly with Scientific Annexes*, # (United Nations Publications, New York).

UNSCEAR (1988).United National Scientific Committee on the Effects of Atomic Radiation. *Sources, Effects and Risks of Ionizing Radiation, 1988 Report to the General Assembly with Annexes* (United Nations Publications, New York).

USP (2004a). U.S. Pharmacopoeia. *Drug Index Volume III. Approved Drug Products and Legal Requirements* (Thomson Healthcare Inc., Stamford, Connecticut).

USP (2004b). U.S. Pharmacopoeia. *Drug Index Volume I. Drug Information for the Health Care Professional* (Thomson Healthcare Inc., Stamford, Connecticut).

VAN DYK, J., BARNETT, R.B., CYGLER, J.E. and SHRAGGE, P.C. (1993). "Commissioning and quality assurance of treatment planning computers," Int. J. Radiat. Oncol. Biol. Phys. **26**(2) 261–273.

WALLACE, A.B. and BUSH, V. (1991), "Management and autopsy of a radioactive cadaver," Aust. Phys. Eng. Sci. Med. **14**(2), 119–124.

WARTERS, R.L., HOFER K.G., HARRIS, C.R. and SMITH, J.M. (1977). "Radionuclide toxicity in cultured mammalian cells: Elucidation of the primary site of radiation damage," Curr. Top. Radiat. Res. Q. **12**(1–4), 389–407.

WELSH, J.S., KENNEDY, A.S. and THOMADSEN, B. (2006). "Selective internal radiation therapy (SIRT) for liver metastases secondary to colorectal adenocarcinoma," Int. J. Radiat. Oncol. Biol. Phys. **66** (Suppl. 2), S62–S73.

WESSELS, B.W. and ROGUS, R.D. (1984). "Radionuclide selection and model absorbed dose calculations for radiolabeled tumor associated antibodies," Med. Phys. **11**(5), 638–645.

WILLIAMSON, J.F. (1988). "Monte Carlo and analytic calculation of absorbed dose near ^{137}Cs intracavitary sources," Int. J. Radiat. Oncol. Biol. Phys. **15**(1), 227–237.

WILLIAMSON, J.F. (1991a). "Practical quality assurance in low-dose rate brachytherapy," pages 139 to 182 in *Proceedings of American College of Medical Physics-Sponsored Symposium on Quality Assurance in Radiotherapy Physics*, Starkswchall, G., Ed. (Medical Physics Publishing Company, Madison, Wisconsin).

WILLIAMSON, J.F. (1991b). "Comparison of measured and calculated dose rates in water near ^{125}I and ^{192}Ir seeds," Med. Phys. **18**(4), 776–778.

WILLIAMSON, J. F. (1994). "Recent advances in brachytherapy dosimetry," in *Radiation Therapy Physics*, Smith, A.R., Ed. (Springer-Verlag, Berlin).

WILLIAMSON, J.F. (1995). "Simulation and source localization procedures for pulsed and high dose-rate brachytherapy," pages 57 to 65 in *Quality Assurance: Activity Special Report No. 7* (Nucletron-Oldelft International B.V., Veenendaal, The Netherlands).

WILLIAMSON, J.F. (1996). "The sievert integral revisited: Evaluation and extension to ^{125}I, ^{169}Yb and ^{192}Ir brachytherapy sources," Int. J. Radiat. Oncol. Biol. Phys. **36**(5), 1239–1250.

WILLIAMSON, J.F. (1998). "Physics of brachytherapy," pages 405 to 468 in *Principles and Practice of Radiation Oncology*, 3rd ed., Perez, C.A. and Brady, L.W., Eds. (J.B. Lippincott Company, Philadelphia).

WILLIAMSON, J.F. and LI, Z. (1995). "Monte Carlo aided dosimetry of the microselectron pulsed and high dose-rate ^{192}Ir sources," Med. Phys. **22**(6), 809–820.

WILLIAMSON, J.F., ANDERSON, L.L., GRIGSBY, P.W., MARTINEZ, A., NATH, R., NEBLETT, D., OLCH, A. and WEAVER, K. (1993). "American Endocurietherapy Society recommendations for specification of brachytherapy source strength," Endocurietherapy/Hyperthermia Oncol. **9**, 1–7.

WILLIAMSON, J.F., EZZELL, G.E., OLCH, A.O. and THOMADSON, B.T. (1994). "Quality assurance for high dose-rate remote afterloading brachytherapy," in *Textbook on High Dose Rate Brachytherapy*, Nag, S., Ed. (Futura Publishing Company, Armonk, New York).

WILLIAMSON, J.F., GRIGSBY, P.W., MEIGOONI, A.S. and TEAGUE, S. (1995). "Clinical physics of pulsed dose-rate remotely-afterloaded brachytherapy," pages 577 to 616 in *Brachytherapy Physics*, Williamson, J.F., Thomadsen, B.T. and Nath, R., Eds. (Medical Physics Publishing Company, Madison, Wisconsin).

WILLIAMSON, J.F., COURSEY, B.M., DEWERD, L.A., HANSON, W.F. and NATH, R. (1998). "Dosimetric perquisites for routine clinical use of new low energy photon interstitial brachytherapy sources," Med. Phys. **25**(12), 2269–2270.

WITZIG, T.E. (2006). "Radioimmunotherapy for B-cell non-Hodgkin's lymphoma," Best Pract. Res. Clin. Haematol. **19**(4), 655–668.

ZANZONICO, P.B. (1997). "Radiation dose to patients and relatives incident to ^{131}I therapy," Thyroid **7**(2), 199–204.

ZANZONICO, P.B. (2000). "Internal radionuclide radiation dosimetry: A review of basic concepts and recent developments," J. Nucl. Med. **41**(2), 297–308.

ZANZONICO, P.B. (2004). "Positron emission tomography: A review of basic principles, scanner design and performance, and current systems," Sem. Nucl. Med. **34**(2), 87–111.

ZANZONICO, P.B. and BECKER, D.V. (1991). "Radiation hazards in children born to mothers exposed to ^{131}I-iodide," pages 189 to 202 in *The Thyroid and Pregnancy*, Beckers, C. and Reinwein, D., Eds. (Schattauer, Stuttgart, Germany).

ZANZONICO, P.B. and HELLER, S. (2000). "The intraoperative gamma probe: Basic principles and choices available," Sem. Nucl. Med. **30**(1), 33–48.

ZANZONICO, P.B., BRILL, A.B. and BECKER, D.V. (1995). "Radiation dosimetry," pages 106 to 134 in *Principles of Nuclear Medicine*, 2nd ed., Buchanan, J., Szabo, Z. and Wagner, H., Eds. (W.B. Saunders, Philadelphia).

ZANZONICO, P.B., BECKER, D. and GOLDSMITH S. (1997). "Release criteria for patients receiving therapeutic amounts of radioactivity: A re-evaluation based on published dosimetry data," J. Nucl. Med. **38**, 229P.

ZANZONICO, P.B., BINKERT, B. and GOLDSMITH, S.J. (1999). "Bremsstrahlung radiation exposure from pure beta-ray emitters," J. Nucl. Med. **40**(6), 1024–1028.

ZANZONICO, P.B., SIEGEL, J.A. and ST. GERMAIN, J. (2000). "A generalized algorithm for determining the time of release and the duration of post-release radiation precautions following radionuclide therapy," Health Phys. **78**(6), 648–659.

The NCRP

The National Council on Radiation Protection and Measurements is a nonprofit corporation chartered by Congress in 1964 to:

1. Collect, analyze, develop and disseminate in the public interest information and recommendations about (a) protection against radiation and (b) radiation measurements, quantities and units, particularly those concerned with radiation protection.
2. Provide a means by which organizations concerned with the scientific and related aspects of radiation protection and of radiation quantities, units and measurements may cooperate for effective utilization of their combined resources, and to stimulate the work of such organizations.
3. Develop basic concepts about radiation quantities, units and measurements, about the application of these concepts, and about radiation protection.
4. Cooperate with the International Commission on Radiological Protection, the International Commission on Radiation Units and Measurements, and other national and international organizations, governmental and private, concerned with radiation quantities, units and measurements and with radiation protection.

The Council is the successor to the unincorporated association of scientists known as the National Committee on Radiation Protection and Measurements and was formed to carry on the work begun by the Committee in 1929.

The participants in the Council's work are the Council members and members of scientific and administrative committees. Council members are selected solely on the basis of their scientific expertise and serve as individuals, not as representatives of any particular organization. The scientific committees, composed of experts having detailed knowledge and competence in the particular area of the committee's interest, draft proposed recommendations. These are then submitted to the full membership of the Council for careful review and approval before being published.

The following comprise the current officers and membership of the Council:

Officers

President	Thomas S. Tenforde
Senior Vice President	Kenneth R. Kase
Secretary and Treasurer	David A. Schauer

Lauriston S. Taylor Lecturers

Patricia W. Durbin (2007) *The Quest for Therapeutic Actinide Chelators*

Robert L. Brent (2006) *Fifty Years of Scientific Research: The Importance of Scholarship and the Influence of Politics and Controversy*

John B. Little (2005) *Nontargeted Effects of Radiation: Implications for Low-Dose Exposures*

Abel J. Gonzalez (2004) *Radiation Protection in the Aftermath of a Terrorist Attack Involving Exposure to Ionizing Radiation*

Charles B. Meinhold (2003) *The Evolution of Radiation Protection: From Erythema to Genetic Risks to Risks of Cancer to ?*

R. Julian Preston (2002) *Developing Mechanistic Data for Incorporation into Cancer Risk Assessment: Old Problems and New Approaches*

Wesley L. Nyborg (2001) *Assuring the Safety of Medical Diagnostic Ultrasound*

S. James Adelstein (2000) *Administered Radioactivity: Unde Venimus Quoque Imus*

Naomi H. Harley (1999) *Back to Background*

Eric J. Hall (1998) *From Chimney Sweeps to Astronauts: Cancer Risks in the Workplace*

William J. Bair (1997) *Radionuclides in the Body: Meeting the Challenge!*

Seymour Abrahamson (1996) *70 Years of Radiation Genetics: Fruit Flies, Mice and Humans*

Albrecht Kellerer (1995) *Certainty and Uncertainty in Radiation Protection*

R.J. Michael Fry (1994) *Mice, Myths and Men*

Warren K. Sinclair (1993) *Science, Radiation Protection and the NCRP*

Edward W. Webster (1992) *Dose and Risk in Diagnostic Radiology: How Big? How Little?*

Victor P. Bond (1991) *When is a Dose Not a Dose?*

J. Newell Stannard (1990) *Radiation Protection and the Internal Emitter Saga*

Arthur C. Upton (1989) *Radiobiology and Radiation Protection: The Past Century and Prospects for the Future*

Bo Lindell (1988) *How Safe is Safe Enough?*

Seymour Jablon (1987) *How to be Quantitative about Radiation Risk Estimates*

Herman P. Schwan (1986) *Biological Effects of Non-ionizing Radiations: Cellular Properties and Interactions*

John H. Harley (1985) *Truth (and Beauty) in Radiation Measurement*

Harald H. Rossi (1984) *Limitation and Assessment in Radiation Protection*

Merril Eisenbud (1983) *The Human Environment—Past, Present and Future*

Eugene L. Saenger (1982) *Ethics, Trade-Offs and Medical Radiation*

James F. Crow (1981) *How Well Can We Assess Genetic Risk? Not Very*

Harold O. Wyckoff (1980) *From "Quantity of Radiation" and "Dose" to "Exposure" and "Absorbed Dose"—An Historical Review*

Hymer L. Friedell (1979) *Radiation Protection—Concepts and Trade Offs*

Sir Edward Pochin (1978) *Why be Quantitative about Radiation Risk Estimates?*

Herbert M. Parker (1977) *The Squares of the Natural Numbers in Radiation Protection*

Currently, the following committees are actively engaged in formulating recommendations:

Program Area Committee 1: Basic Criteria, Epidemiology, Radiobiology, and Risk
    SC 1-8 Risk to Thyroid from Ionizing Radiation
    SC 1-13 Impact of Individual Susceptibility and Previous Radiation Exposure on Radiation Risk for Astronauts
    SC 1-15 Radiation Safety in NASA Lunar Missions'
    SC 1-17 Second Cancers and Cardiopulmonary Effects After Radiotherapy
    SC 85 Risk of Lung Cancer from Radon
Program Area Committee 2: Operational Radiation Safety
    SC 2-3 Radiation Safety Issues for Image-Guided Interventional Medical Procedures
    SC 2-4 Self Assessment of Radiation Safety Programs
    SC 46-17 Radiation Protection in Educational Institutions
Program Area Committee 3: Nonionizing Radiation
Program Area Committee 4: Radiation Protection in Medicine
    SC 4-1 Management of Persons Contaminated with Radionuclides
    SC 4-2 Population Monitoring and Decontamination Following a Nuclear/ Radiological Incident
Program Area Committee 5: Environmental Radiation and Radioactive Waste Issues
    SC 64-22 Design of Effective Effluent and Environmental Monitoring Programs
Program Area Committee 6: Radiation Measurements and Dosimetry
    SC 6-1 Uncertainties in the Measurement and Dosimetry of External Radiation Sources
    SC 6-2 Radiation Exposure of the U.S. Population
    SC 6-3 Uncertainties in Internal Radiation Dosimetry
    SC 6-4 Fundamental Principles of Dose Reconstruction
    SC 6-5 Radiation Protection and Measurement Issues Related to Cargo Scanning with High-Energy X Rays Produced by Accelerators
    SC 6-6 Skin Doses from Dermal Contamination
    SC 6-7 Evaluation of Inhalation Doses in Scenarios Involving Resuspension by Nuclear Detonations at the Nevada Test Site

In recognition of its responsibility to facilitate and stimulate cooperation among organizations concerned with the scientific and related aspects of radiation protection and measurement, the Council has created a category of NCRP Collaborating Organizations. Organizations or groups of organizations that are national or international in scope and are concerned with scientific problems involving radiation quantities, units, measurements and effects, or radiation protection may be admitted to collaborating status by the Council. Collaborating Organizations provide a means by which NCRP can gain input into its activities from a wider segment of society. At the same time, the relationships with the Collaborating Organizations facilitate wider dissemination of information about the Council's activities, interests and concerns. Collaborating Organizations have the opportunity to comment on draft reports (at the time that these are submitted to the members of the Council). This is intended to capitalize on the fact that Collaborating Organizations are in an excellent position to both contribute to the identification of what needs to be treated in NCRP reports and to identify problems that might result from proposed recommendations. The present Collaborating Organizations with which NCRP maintains liaison are as follows:

American Academy of Dermatology
American Academy of Environmental Engineers
American Academy of Health Physics
American Association of Physicists in Medicine
American College of Medical Physics
American College of Nuclear Physicians
American College of Occupational and Environmental Medicine
American College of Radiology
American Conference of Governmental Industrial Hygienists
American Dental Association
American Industrial Hygiene Association
American Institute of Ultrasound in Medicine
American Medical Association
American Nuclear Society
American Pharmaceutical Association
American Podiatric Medical Association
American Public Health Association
American Radium Society
American Roentgen Ray Society
American Society for Therapeutic Radiology and Oncology
American Society of Emergency Radiology
American Society of Health-System Pharmacists
American Society of Radiologic Technologists
Association of Educators in Imaging and Radiological Sciences
Association of University Radiologists
Bioelectromagnetics Society
Campus Radiation Safety Officers
College of American Pathologists
Conference of Radiation Control Program Directors, Inc.
Council on Radionuclides and Radiopharmaceuticals
Defense Threat Reduction Agency
Electric Power Research Institute
Federal Communications Commission
Federal Emergency Management Agency
Genetics Society of America
Health Physics Society
Institute of Electrical and Electronics Engineers, Inc.
Institute of Nuclear Power Operations
International Brotherhood of Electrical Workers
National Aeronautics and Space Administration
National Association of Environmental Professionals
National Center for Environmental Health/Agency for Toxic Substances
National Electrical Manufacturers Association
National Institute for Occupational Safety and Health
National Institute of Standards and Technology
Nuclear Energy Institute

Office of Science and Technology Policy
Paper, Allied-Industrial, Chemical and Energy Workers International
Union
Product Stewardship Institute
Radiation Research Society
Radiological Society of North America
Society for Cardiovascular Angiography and Interventions
Society for Risk Analysis
Society of Chairmen of Academic Radiology Departments
Society of Interventional Radiology
Society of Nuclear Medicine
Society of Radiologists in Ultrasound
Society of Skeletal Radiology
U.S. Air Force
U.S. Army
U.S. Coast Guard
U.S. Department of Energy
U.S. Department of Housing and Urban Development
U.S. Department of Labor
U.S. Department of Transportation
U.S. Environmental Protection Agency
U.S. Navy
U.S. Nuclear Regulatory Commission
U.S. Public Health Service
Utility Workers Union of America

NCRP has found its relationships with these organizations to be extremely valuable to continued progress in its program.

Another aspect of the cooperative efforts of NCRP relates to the Special Liaison relationships established with various governmental organizations that have an interest in radiation protection and measurements. This liaison relationship provides: (1) an opportunity for participating organizations to designate an individual to provide liaison between the organization and NCRP; (2) that the individual designated will receive copies of draft NCRP reports (at the time that these are submitted to the members of the Council) with an invitation to comment, but not vote; and (3) that new NCRP efforts might be discussed with liaison individuals as appropriate, so that they might have an opportunity to make suggestions on new studies and related matters. The following organizations participate in the Special Liaison Program:

Australian Radiation Laboratory
Bundesamt fur Strahlenschutz (Germany)
Canadian Nuclear Safety Commission
Central Laboratory for Radiological Protection (Poland)
China Institute for Radiation Protection
Commissariat a l'Energie Atomique (France)
Commonwealth Scientific Instrumentation Research Organization
(Australia)
European Commission
Health Council of the Netherlands
Health Protection Agency

International Commission on Non-ionizing Radiation Protection
International Commission on Radiation Units and Measurements
Japan Radiation Council
Korea Institute of Nuclear Safety
Russian Scientific Commission on Radiation Protection
South African Forum for Radiation Protection
World Association of Nuclear Operators
World Health Organization, Radiation and Environmental Health

NCRP values highly the participation of these organizations in the Special Liaison Program.

The Council also benefits significantly from the relationships established pursuant to the Corporate Sponsor's Program. The program facilitates the interchange of information and ideas and corporate sponsors provide valuable fiscal support for the Council's program. This developing program currently includes the following Corporate Sponsors:

3M
Duke Energy Corporation
GE Healthcare
Global Dosimetry Solutions, Inc.
Landauer, Inc.
Nuclear Energy Institute

The Council's activities have been made possible by the voluntary contribution of time and effort by its members and participants and the generous support of the following organizations:

3M Health Physics Services
Agfa Corporation
Alfred P. Sloan Foundation
Alliance of American Insurers
American Academy of Dermatology
American Academy of Health Physics
American Academy of Oral and Maxillofacial Radiology
American Association of Physicists in Medicine
American Cancer Society
American College of Medical Physics
American College of Nuclear Physicians
American College of Occupational and Environmental Medicine
American College of Radiology
American College of Radiology Foundation
American Dental Association
American Healthcare Radiology Administrators
American Industrial Hygiene Association
American Insurance Services Group
American Medical Association
American Nuclear Society
American Osteopathic College of Radiology
American Podiatric Medical Association
American Public Health Association

American Radium Society
American Roentgen Ray Society
American Society of Radiologic Technologists
American Society for Therapeutic Radiology and Oncology
American Veterinary Medical Association
American Veterinary Radiology Society
Association of Educators in Radiological Sciences, Inc.
Association of University Radiologists
Battelle Memorial Institute
Canberra Industries, Inc.
Chem Nuclear Systems
Center for Devices and Radiological Health
College of American Pathologists
Committee on Interagency Radiation Research and Policy Coordination
Commonwealth Edison
Commonwealth of Pennsylvania
Consolidated Edison
Consumers Power Company
Council on Radionuclides and Radiopharmaceuticals
Defense Nuclear Agency
Defense Threat Reduction Agency
Eastman Kodak Company
Edison Electric Institute
Edward Mallinckrodt, Jr. Foundation
EG&G Idaho, Inc.
Electric Power Research Institute
Electromagnetic Energy Association
Federal Emergency Management Agency
Florida Institute of Phosphate Research
Florida Power Corporation
Fuji Medical Systems, U.S.A., Inc.
Genetics Society of America
Global Dosimetry Solutions
Health Effects Research Foundation (Japan)
Health Physics Society
ICN Biomedicals, Inc.
Institute of Nuclear Power Operations
James Picker Foundation
Martin Marietta Corporation
Motorola Foundation
National Aeronautics and Space Administration
National Association of Photographic Manufacturers
National Cancer Institute
National Electrical Manufacturers Association
National Institute of Standards and Technology
New York Power Authority
Philips Medical Systems
Picker International
Public Service Electric and Gas Company
Radiation Research Society

Initial funds for publication of NCRP reports were provided by a grant from the James Picker Foundation.

NCRP seeks to promulgate information and recommendations based on leading scientific judgment on matters of radiation protection and measurement and to foster cooperation among organizations concerned with these matters. These efforts are intended to serve the public interest and the Council welcomes comments and suggestions on its reports or activities.

NCRP Publications

NCRP publications can be obtained online in both hard- and soft-copy (downloadable PDF) formats at http://NCRPpublications.org. Professional societies can arrange for discounts for their members by contacting NCRP. Additional information on NCRP publications may be obtained from the NCRP website (http://NCRPonline.org) or by telephone (800-229-2652, ext. 25) and fax (301-907-8768). The mailing address is:

NCRP Publications
7910 Woodmont Avenue
Suite 400
Bethesda, MD 20814-3095

Abstracts of NCRP reports published since 1980, abstracts of all NCRP commentaries, and the text of all NCRP statements are available at the NCRP website. Currently available publications are listed below.

NCRP Reports

No.   Title

8   *Control and Removal of Radioactive Contamination in Laboratories* (1951)
22   *Maximum Permissible Body Burdens and Maximum Permissible Concentrations of Radionuclides in Air and in Water for Occupational Exposure* (1959) [includes Addendum 1 issued in August 1963]
25   *Measurement of Absorbed Dose of Neutrons, and of Mixtures of Neutrons and Gamma Rays* (1961)
27   *Stopping Powers for Use with Cavity Chambers* (1961)
30   *Safe Handling of Radioactive Materials* (1964)
32   *Radiation Protection in Educational Institutions* (1966)
35   *Dental X-Ray Protection* (1970)
36   *Radiation Protection in Veterinary Medicine* (1970)
37   *Precautions in the Management of Patients Who Have Received Therapeutic Amounts of Radionuclides* (1970)
38   *Protection Against Neutron Radiation* (1971)
40   *Protection Against Radiation from Brachytherapy Sources* (1972)
41   *Specification of Gamma-Ray Brachytherapy Sources* (1974)
42   *Radiological Factors Affecting Decision-Making in a Nuclear Attack* (1974)
44   *Krypton-85 in the Atmosphere—Accumulation, Biological Significance, and Control Technology* (1975)
46   *Alpha-Emitting Particles in Lungs* (1975)

117 *Research Needs for Radiation Protection* (1993)
118 *Radiation Protection in the Mineral Extraction Industry* (1993)
119 *A Practical Guide to the Determination of Human Exposure to Radiofrequency Fields* (1993)
120 *Dose Control at Nuclear Power Plants* (1994)
121 *Principles and Application of Collective Dose in Radiation Protection* (1995)
122 *Use of Personal Monitors to Estimate Effective Dose Equivalent and Effective Dose to Workers for External Exposure to Low-LET Radiation* (1995)
123 *Screening Models for Releases of Radionuclides to Atmosphere, Surface Water, and Ground* (1996)
124 *Sources and Magnitude of Occupational and Public Exposures from Nuclear Medicine Procedures* (1996)
125 *Deposition, Retention and Dosimetry of Inhaled Radioactive Substances* (1997)
126 *Uncertainties in Fatal Cancer Risk Estimates Used in Radiation Protection* (1997)
127 *Operational Radiation Safety Program* (1998)
128 *Radionuclide Exposure of the Embryo / Fetus* (1998)
129 *Recommended Screening Limits for Contaminated Surface Soil and Review of Factors Relevant to Site-Specific Studies* (1999)
130 *Biological Effects and Exposure Limits for "Hot Particles"* (1999)
131 *Scientific Basis for Evaluating the Risks to Populations from Space Applications of Plutonium* (2001)
132 *Radiation Protection Guidance for Activities in Low-Earth Orbit* (2000)
133 *Radiation Protection for Procedures Performed Outside the Radiology Department* (2000)
134 *Operational Radiation Safety Training* (2000)
135 *Liver Cancer Risk from Internally-Deposited Radionuclides* (2001)
136 *Evaluation of the Linear-Nonthreshold Dose-Response Model for Ionizing Radiation* (2001)
137 *Fluence-Based and Microdosimetric Event-Based Methods for Radiation Protection in Space* (2001)
138 *Management of Terrorist Events Involving Radioactive Material* (2001)
139 *Risk-Based Classification of Radioactive and Hazardous Chemical Wastes* (2002)
140 *Exposure Criteria for Medical Diagnostic Ultrasound: II. Criteria Based on all Known Mechanisms* (2002)
141 *Managing Potentially Radioactive Scrap Metal* (2002)
142 *Operational Radiation Safety Program for Astronauts in Low-Earth Orbit: A Basic Framework* (2002)
143 *Management Techniques for Laboratories and Other Small Institutional Generators to Minimize Off-Site Disposal of Low-Level Radioactive Waste* (2003)
144 *Radiation Protection for Particle Accelerator Facilities* (2003)
145 *Radiation Protection in Dentistry* (2003)

146 *Approaches to Risk Management in Remediation of Radioactively Contaminated Sites* (2004)
147 *Structural Shielding Design for Medical X-Ray Imaging Facilities* (2004)
148 *Radiation Protection in Veterinary Medicine* (2004)
149 *A Guide to Mammography and Other Breast Imaging Procedures* (2004)
150 *Extrapolation of Radiation-Induced Cancer Risks from Nonhuman Experimental Systems to Humans* (2005)
151 *Structural Shielding Design and Evaluation for Megavoltage X- and Gamma-Ray Radiotherapy Facilities* (2005)
152 *Performance Assessment of Near-Surface Facilities for Disposal of Low-Level Radioactive Waste* (2005)
153 *Information Needed to Make Radiation Protection Recommendations for Space Missions Beyond Low-Earth Orbit* (2006)
154 *Cesium-137 in the Environment: Radioecology and Approaches to Assessment and Management* (2006)
155 *Management of Radionuclide Therapy Patients* (2006)

Binders for NCRP reports are available. Two sizes make it possible to collect into small binders the "old series" of reports (NCRP Reports Nos. 8–30) and into large binders the more recent publications (NCRP Reports Nos. 32–155). Each binder will accommodate from five to seven reports. The binders carry the identification "NCRP Reports" and come with label holders which permit the user to attach labels showing the reports contained in each binder.

The following bound sets of NCRP reports are also available:

Volume I. NCRP Reports Nos. 8, 22
Volume II. NCRP Reports Nos. 23, 25, 27, 30
Volume III. NCRP Reports Nos. 32, 35, 36, 37
Volume IV. NCRP Reports Nos. 38, 40, 41
Volume V. NCRP Reports Nos. 42, 44, 46
Volume VI. NCRP Reports Nos. 47, 49, 50, 51
Volume VII. NCRP Reports Nos. 52, 53, 54, 55, 57
Volume VIII. NCRP Report No. 58
Volume IX. NCRP Reports Nos. 59, 60, 61, 62, 63
Volume X. NCRP Reports Nos. 64, 65, 66, 67
Volume XI. NCRP Reports Nos. 68, 69, 70, 71, 72
Volume XII. NCRP Reports Nos. 73, 74, 75, 76
Volume XIII. NCRP Reports Nos. 77, 78, 79, 80
Volume XIV. NCRP Reports Nos. 81, 82, 83, 84, 85
Volume XV. NCRP Reports Nos. 86, 87, 88, 89
Volume XVI. NCRP Reports Nos. 90, 91, 92, 93
Volume XVII. NCRP Reports Nos. 94, 95, 96, 97
Volume XVIII. NCRP Reports Nos. 98, 99, 100
Volume XIX. NCRP Reports Nos. 101, 102, 103, 104
Volume XX. NCRP Reports Nos. 105, 106, 107, 108
Volume XXI. NCRP Reports Nos. 109, 110, 111
Volume XXII. NCRP Reports Nos. 112, 113, 114
Volume XXIII. NCRP Reports Nos. 115, 116, 117, 118

Volume XXIV. NCRP Reports Nos. 119, 120, 121, 122
Volume XXV. NCRP Report No. 123I and 123II
Volume XXVI. NCRP Reports Nos. 124, 125, 126, 127
Volume XXVII. NCRP Reports Nos. 128, 129, 130
Volume XXVIII. NCRP Reports Nos. 131, 132, 133
Volume XXIX. NCRP Reports Nos. 134, 135, 136, 137
Volume XXX. NCRP Reports Nos. 138, 139
Volume XXXI. NCRP Report No. 140
Volume XXXII. NCRP Reports Nos. 141, 142, 143
Volume XXXIII. NCRP Report No. 144
Volume XXXIV. NCRP Reports Nos. 145, 146, 147
Volume XXXV. NCRP Reports Nos. 148, 149
Volume XXXVI. NCRP Reports Nos. 150, 151, 152

(Titles of the individual reports contained in each volume are given previously.)

NCRP Commentaries

No.   Title

1   *Krypton-85 in the Atmosphere—With Specific Reference to the Public Health Significance of the Proposed Controlled Release at Three Mile Island* (1980)

4   *Guidelines for the Release of Waste Water from Nuclear Facilities with Special Reference to the Public Health Significance of the Proposed Release of Treated Waste Waters at Three Mile Island* (1987)

5   *Review of the Publication, Living Without Landfills* (1989)

6   *Radon Exposure of the U.S. Population—Status of the Problem (1991)*

7   *Misadministration of Radioactive Material in Medicine—Scientific Background* (1991)

8   *Uncertainty in NCRP Screening Models Relating to Atmospheric Transport, Deposition and Uptake by Humans* (1993)

9   *Considerations Regarding the Unintended Radiation Exposure of the Embryo, Fetus or Nursing Child* (1994)

10 *Advising the Public about Radiation Emergencies: A Document for Public Comment* (1994)

11 *Dose Limits for Individuals Who Receive Exposure from Radionuclide Therapy Patients* (1995)

12 *Radiation Exposure and High-Altitude Flight* (1995)

13 *An Introduction to Efficacy in Diagnostic Radiology and Nuclear Medicine (Justification of Medical Radiation Exposure)* (1995)

14 *A Guide for Uncertainty Analysis in Dose and Risk Assessments Related to Environmental Contamination* (1996)

15 *Evaluating the Reliability of Biokinetic and Dosimetric Models and Parameters Used to Assess Individual Doses for Risk Assessment Purposes* (1998)

16 *Screening of Humans for Security Purposes Using Ionizing Radiation Scanning Systems* (2003)

17 *Pulsed Fast Neutron Analysis System Used in Security Surveillance* (2003)

18   *Biological Effects of Modulated Radiofrequency Fields* (2003)
19   *Key Elements of Preparing Emergency Responders for Nuclear and Radiological Terrorism* (2005)

Proceedings of the Annual Meeting

No.   Title

1   *Perceptions of Risk,* Proceedings of the Fifteenth Annual Meeting held on March 14-15, 1979 (including Taylor Lecture No. 3) (1980)

3   *Critical Issues in Setting Radiation Dose Limits*, Proceedings of the Seventeenth Annual Meeting held on April 8-9, 1981 (including Taylor Lecture No. 5) (1982)

4   *Radiation Protection and New Medical Diagnostic Approaches,* Proceedings of the Eighteenth Annual Meeting held on April 6-7, 1982 (including Taylor Lecture No. 6) (1983)

5   *Environmental Radioactivity,* Proceedings of the Nineteenth Annual Meeting held on April 6-7, 1983 (including Taylor Lecture No. 7) (1983)

6   *Some Issues Important in Developing Basic Radiation Protection Recommendations*, Proceedings of the Twentieth Annual Meeting held on April 4-5, 1984 (including Taylor Lecture No. 8) (1985)

7   *Radioactive Waste*, Proceedings of the Twenty-first Annual Meeting held on April 3-4, 1985 (including Taylor Lecture No. 9)(1986)

8   *Nonionizing Electromagnetic Radiations and Ultrasound,* Proceedings of the Twenty-second Annual Meeting held on April 2-3, 1986 (including Taylor Lecture No. 10) (1988)

9   *New Dosimetry at Hiroshima and Nagasaki and Its Implications for Risk Estimates*, Proceedings of the Twenty-third Annual Meeting held on April 8-9, 1987 (including Taylor Lecture No. 11) (1988)

10   *Radon*, Proceedings of the Twenty-fourth Annual Meeting held on March 30-31, 1988 (including Taylor Lecture No. 12) (1989)

11   *Radiation Protection Today—The NCRP at Sixty Years*, Proceedings of the Twenty-fifth Annual Meeting held on April 5-6, 1989 (including Taylor Lecture No. 13) (1990)

12   *Health and Ecological Implications of Radioactively Contaminated Environments*, Proceedings of the Twenty-sixth Annual Meeting held on April 4-5, 1990 (including Taylor Lecture No. 14) (1991)

13   *Genes, Cancer and Radiation Protection,* Proceedings of the Twenty-seventh Annual Meeting held on April 3-4, 1991 (including Taylor Lecture No. 15) (1992)

14   *Radiation Protection in Medicine,* Proceedings of the Twenty-eighth Annual Meeting held on April 1-2, 1992 (including Taylor Lecture No. 16) (1993)

15   *Radiation Science and Societal Decision Making,* Proceedings of the Twenty-ninth Annual Meeting held on April 7-8, 1993 (including Taylor Lecture No. 17) (1994)

16   *Extremely-Low-Frequency Electromagnetic Fields: Issues in Biological Effects and Public Health*, Proceedings of the Thirtieth Annual Meeting held on April 6-7, 1994 (not published).

17 *Environmental Dose Reconstruction and Risk Implications*, Proceedings of the Thirty-first Annual Meeting held on April 12-13, 1995 (including Taylor Lecture No. 19) (1996)

18 *Implications of New Data on Radiation Cancer Risk*, Proceedings of the Thirty-second Annual Meeting held on April 3-4, 1996 (including Taylor Lecture No. 20) (1997)

19 *The Effects of Pre- and Postconception Exposure to Radiation*, Proceedings of the Thirty-third Annual Meeting held on April 2-3, 1997, Teratology **59**, 181–317 (1999)

20 *Cosmic Radiation Exposure of Airline Crews, Passengers and Astronauts*, Proceedings of the Thirty-fourth Annual Meeting held on April 1-2, 1998, Health Phys. **79**, 466–613 (2000)

21 *Radiation Protection in Medicine: Contemporary Issues*, Proceedings of the Thirty-fifth Annual Meeting held on April 7-8, 1999 (including Taylor Lecture No. 23) (1999)

22 *Ionizing Radiation Science and Protection in the 21st Century*, Proceedings of the Thirty-sixth Annual Meeting held on April 5-6, 2000, Health Phys. **80**, 317–402 (2001)

23 *Fallout from Atmospheric Nuclear Tests—Impact on Science and Society*, Proceedings of the Thirty-seventh Annual Meeting held on April 4-5, 2001, Health Phys. **82**, 573–748 (2002)

24 *Where the New Biology Meets Epidemiology: Impact on Radiation Risk Estimates*, Proceedings of the Thirty-eighth Annual Meeting held on April 10-11, 2002, Health Phys. **85**, 1–108 (2003)

25 *Radiation Protection at the Beginning of the 21st Century–A Look Forward*, Proceedings of the Thirty-ninth Annual Meeting held on April 9–10, 2003, Health Phys. **87**, 237–319 (2004)

26 *Advances in Consequence Management for Radiological Terrorism Events*, Proceedings of the Fortieth Annual Meeting held on April 14–15, 2004, Health Phys. **89**, 415–588 (2005)

27 *Managing the Disposition of Low-Activity Radioactive Materials*, Proceedings of the Forty-first Annual Meeting held on March 30–31, 2005, Health Phys. **91**, 413–536 (2006)

Lauriston S. Taylor Lectures

No.   Title

1 *The Squares of the Natural Numbers in Radiation Protection by* Herbert M. Parker (1977)

2 *Why be Quantitative about Radiation Risk Estimates?* by Sir Edward Pochin (1978)

3 *Radiation Protection—Concepts and Trade Offs* by Hymer L. Friedell (1979) [available also in *Perceptions of Risk*, see above]

4 *From "Quantity of Radiation" and "Dose" to "Exposure" and "Absorbed Dose"—An Historical Review* by Harold O. Wyckoff (1980)

5 *How Well Can We Assess Genetic Risk? Not Very* by James F. Crow (1981) [available also in *Critical Issues in Setting Radiation Dose Limits*, see above]

6   *Ethics, Trade-offs and Medical Radiation* by Eugene L. Saenger (1982) [available also in *Radiation Protection and New Medical Diagnostic Approaches*, see above]

7   *The Human Environment—Past, Present and Future* by Merril Eisenbud (1983) [available also in *Environmental Radioactivity*, see above]

8   *Limitation and Assessment in Radiation Protection* by Harald H. Rossi (1984) [available also in *Some Issues Important in Developing Basic Radiation Protection Recommendations*, see above]

9   *Truth (and Beauty) in Radiation Measurement* by John H. Harley (1985) [available also in *Radioactive Waste*, see above]

10 *Biological Effects of Non-ionizing Radiations: Cellular Properties and Interactions* by Herman P. Schwan (1987) [available also in *Nonionizing Electromagnetic Radiations and Ultrasound*, see above]

11 *How to be Quantitative about Radiation Risk Estimates* by Seymour Jablon (1988) [available also in *New Dosimetry at Hiroshima and Nagasaki and its Implications for Risk Estimates*, see above]

12 *How Safe is Safe Enough?* by Bo Lindell (1988) [available also in *Radon*, see above]

13 *Radiobiology and Radiation Protection: The Past Century and Prospects for the Future* by Arthur C. Upton (1989) [available also in *Radiation Protection Today*, see above]

14 *Radiation Protection and the Internal Emitter Saga* by J. Newell Stannard (1990) [available also in *Health and Ecological Implications of Radioactively Contaminated Environments*, see above]

15 *When is a Dose Not a Dose?* by Victor P. Bond (1992) [available also in *Genes, Cancer and Radiation Protection*, see above]

16 *Dose and Risk in Diagnostic Radiology: How Big? How Little?* by Edward W. Webster (1992) [available also in *Radiation Protection in Medicine*, see above]

17 *Science, Radiation Protection and the NCRP* by Warren K. Sinclair (1993) [available also in *Radiation Science and Societal Decision Making*, see above]

18 *Mice, Myths and Men* by R.J. Michael Fry (1995)

19 *Certainty and Uncertainty in Radiation Research* by Albrecht M. Kellerer. Health Phys. **69**, 446–453 (1995)

20 *70 Years of Radiation Genetics: Fruit Flies, Mice and Humans* by Seymour Abrahamson. Health Phys. **71**, 624–633 (1996)

21 *Radionuclides in the Body: Meeting the Challenge* by William J. Bair. Health Phys. **73**, 423–432 (1997)

22 *From Chimney Sweeps to Astronauts: Cancer Risks in the Work Place* by Eric J. Hall. Health Phys. **75**, 357–366 (1998)

23 *Back to Background: Natural Radiation and Radioactivity Exposed* by Naomi H. Harley. Health Phys. **79**, 121–128 (2000)

24 *Administered Radioactivity: Unde Venimus Quoque Imus* by S. James Adelstein. Health Phys. **80**, 317–324 (2001)

25 *Assuring the Safety of Medical Diagnostic Ultrasound* by Wesley L. Nyborg. Health Phys. **82**, 578–587 (2002)

26 *Developing Mechanistic Data for Incorporation into Cancer and Genetic Risk Assessments: Old Problems and New Approaches* by R. Julian Preston. Health Phys. **85**, 4–12 (2003)

27 *The Evolution of Radiation Protection–From Erythema to Genetic Risks to Risks of Cancer to ?* by Charles B. Meinhold, Health Phys. **87**, 240–248 (2004)

28 *Radiation Protection in the Aftermath of a Terrorist Attack Involving Exposure to Ionizing Radiation* by Abel J. Gonzalez, Health Phys. **89**, 418–446 (2005)

29 *Nontargeted Effects of Radiation: Implications for Low Dose Exposures* by John B. Little, Health Phys. **91**, 416–426 (2006)

Symposium Proceedings

No.   Title

1 *The Control of Exposure of the Public to Ionizing Radiation in the Event of Accident or Attack*, Proceedings of a Symposium held April 27-29, 1981 (1982)

2 *Radioactive and Mixed Waste—Risk as a Basis for Waste Classification,* Proceedings of a Symposium held November 9, 1994 (1995)

3 *Acceptability of Risk from Radiation—Application to Human Space Flight,* Proceedings of a Symposium held May 29, 1996 (1997)

4 *21st Century Biodosimetry: Quantifying the Past and Predicting the Future*, Proceedings of a Symposium held February 22, 2001, Radiat. Prot. Dosim. **97**(1), (2001)

5 *National Conference on Dose Reduction in CT, with an Emphasis on Pediatric Patients*, Summary of a Symposium held November 6-7, 2002, Am. J. Roentgenol. **181**(2), 321–339 (2003)

NCRP Statements

No.   Title

1 "Blood Counts, Statement of the National Committee on Radiation Protection," Radiology **63**, 428 (1954)

2 "Statements on Maximum Permissible Dose from Television Receivers and Maximum Permissible Dose to the Skin of the Whole Body," Am. J. Roentgenol., Radium Ther. and Nucl. Med. **84**, 152 (1960) and Radiology **75**, 122 (1960)

3 *X-Ray Protection Standards for Home Television Receivers, Interim Statement of the National Council on Radiation Protection and Measurements* (1968)

4 *Specification of Units of Natural Uranium and Natural Thorium, Statement of the National Council on Radiation Protection and Measurements* (1973)

5 *NCRP Statement on Dose Limit for Neutrons* (1980)

6 *Control of Air Emissions of Radionuclides* (1984)

7 *The Probability That a Particular Malignancy May Have Been Caused by a Specified Irradiation* (1992)

8 *The Application of ALARA for Occupational Exposures* (1999)

9   *Extension of the Skin Dose Limit for Hot Particles to Other External Sources of Skin Irradiation* (2001)
10 *Recent Applications of the NCRP Public Dose Limit Recommendation for Ionizing Radiation* (2004)

Other Documents

The following documents were published outside of the NCRP report, commentary and statement series:

Somatic Radiation Dose for the General Population, Report of the Ad Hoc Committee of the National Council on Radiation Protection and Measurements, 6 May 1959, Science **131** (3399), February 19, 482–486 (1960)

Dose Effect Modifying Factors in Radiation Protection, Report of Subcommittee M-4 (Relative Biological Effectiveness) of the National Council on Radiation Protection and Measurements, Report BNL 50073 (T-471) (1967) Brookhaven National Laboratory (National Technical Information Service, Springfield, Virginia)

Residential Radon Exposure and Lung Cancer Risk: Commentary on Cohen's County-Based Study, Health Phys. **87**(6), 656–658 (2004)

Index